The 2027 Chiropractic Textbook

Volume 1

Claude Lessard, D.C.

© 2023

Dr. Claude Lessard

Dr. Claude Lessard

DEDICATION

TO THOM GELARDI, D.C.

Thousands of chiropractors under the tutelage of Dr. Thom Gelardi have learned and grown as a result of his untiring dedication to chiropractic and its community. Countless lives have been and continue to be enhanced by his unswerving commitment to chiropractic's central idea, the role of vertebral subluxation and its core values, namely, its philosophy, science, and art.

His courage and gifted leadership in continuously maintaining that the process of locating, analyzing, and facilitating the correction of the vertebral subluxation is the sole responsibility of the chiropractor deserves our adherence and protection in order to preserve and promote the sacred trust of chiropractic.

To honor his contribution to the chiropractic profession over the span of some seventy years and for his devotion to the legacy of D.D. and B.J. Palmer, it is with immense gratitude that Volume 1 of The 2027 Chiropractic Textbook is dedicated to Thom A. Gelardi, D.C.

TABLE OF CONTENTS

Dr. Claude Lessard

PREFACE

This is a series of four academic volumes to be studied as part of the chiropractic curriculum for the student to learn chiropractic and graduate as a chiropractor. It is the rectified version of its original precursor, *"CHIROPRACTIC TEXT BOOK"* written by Dr. Ralph W. Stephenson in 1927. Portions of the text are taken directly from the original and updated with NEW knowledge constructed from NEW information of the last hundred years. The same building blocks of chiropractic are refashioned into a contemporary context that includes 130 years of continuous discoveries. Credit is given to Dr. D.D. Palmer, Dr. B.J. Palmer, and Dr. R.W. Stephenson. We all stand on their shoulders as we move forward.

I applied to Sherman College in December of 1973. I was first introduced to the founder of Sherman College, Dr. Thom Gelardi, during the orientation day. Over the years, Dr. Gelardi and I developed a close relationship. After hundreds of hours of conversation, it was at his suggestion, in the summer of 2021 that I undertook the task of rewriting the chiropractic textbook.

I owe much to Dr. Reggie Gold for facilitating the formation of my chiropractic mind and for always encouraging me to THINK and THINK and THINK. I am grateful to Reggie for his constant challenges that stretched me to this day to grasp the unadulterated aspect of the exclusivity of the chiropractic objective.

I have no doubt that without the constant affirmation, encouragement, and deep friendship of Dr. Joseph Strauss this textbook could never have been rewritten.

With heartfelt gratitude, I thank James Healey, D.C. for continuously being my devil's advocate, asking the questions that provide a needed accuracy check to my musings.

Thank you to Dr. Tom Gregory for his steady listening and comments on the accuracy of the text.

Thank you to Dr. Judy Campenale for spending many long hours editing my French Canadian Anglo Saxon writing style into a comprehensive academic text.

Thank you to Dr. Jack Bourla whose insights help to clarify some of the more difficult concepts to understand.

Thank you to Amanda Janiec for overseeing the entire project and making it possible.

Finally, to the one and only person who saw me through it all, Sara, my spouse of fifty years without whom I could not be the person that I am today. I love you Sara.

These volumes are simply "The Chiropractic Text Book" updated and re-contextualized. The instructions contained therein are further developed from the original concepts of the founder of chiropractic, Dr. Daniel David Palmer, and his son, the developer of chiropractic, Dr. Bartlett Joshua Palmer. Within these volumes, I hope to falsify and deconstruct the theistic and anthropomorphic characters given to some of chiropractic's scientific principles and scientific laws in those early days, namely universal intelligence and innate intelligence. Those chiropractic concepts are then reconstructed on the solid bedrock of the testable and verifiable principles of chiropractic's basic science; they include new information acquired since 1927 that dictates the chiropractic objective. Theses four volumes contain NEW knowledge that has been discovered and constructed within the past 100 years, NEW information that was unavailable from 1895 to 1927. They cover the philosophy, the science, and the art of chiropractic. They are intended to be a further study of chiropractic, developed to

CARRY ON the genius of our predecessors, D.D. and B.J. Palmer; they are designed to convey more precisely "WHAT" chiropractic is, "HOW" to apply its scientific principles, and the **hard to vary** explanation of "WHY" chiropractic is an evolutionary humanitarian approach to EVERY experience of life, not just the experience of health. These volumes comprise error corrections that are necessary for the student to obtain an assured confidence in the chiropractic objective including its universal value. They honor, yet modernize, this significant discovery and the greater understanding of its necessary and humanitarian service to the world. It was Joseph B. Strauss, D.C. who wrote in 2002, "I do not believe that you can truly understand chiropractic philosophy without studying Stephenson. There are truths within and errors that need to be seen and understood for any student to ever begin to reach a level of comprehension of chiropractic as it was and is today."[1] Students are encouraged to study Stephenson's textbook of 1927, ALL of the Strauss' Blue Books, and the two Blue Books that I have personally authored, *A New Look at Chiropractic's Basic Science* and *Timed Out: Chiropractic*.

It is the hope that the truths and error corrections contained within the pages of these volumes will inform and inspire future generations of chiropractors so that they can make an informed choice in constructing their professional mission. Based on these studies, it is clear that the sole aim of the chiropractic objective is the restoration of normal transmission of innate impulses through the location, analysis, and the facilitation of the correction of vertebral subluxations for a normal transmission of innate impulses. PERIOD.

These texts have been written for educational instruction. They are divided into Volume One (First Year Chiropractic Text), Volume Two (Second Year Chiropractic Text), Volume Three (Third Year Chiropractic Text), and Volume Four (Fourth Year Chiropractic Text). Following the original layout of Stephenson's allowing for the integral comparison of topics. There are questions for review that are intended to help the student THINK and "internalize" the value of chiropractic, and raise inquiry to test any of its 33 scientific principles in order to verify or falsify any of them. The student is urged to become familiar with the unique chiropractic lexicon at the beginning of every volume in order to properly understand the meaning of those terms that will undoubtedly assist the study of the text. Hopefully, these four volumes of the updated chiropractic textbook will encourage future chiropractors to CARRY ON and further develop chiropractic, that will include NEW knowledge, insights, and error corrections into the third millennium and forever more.

---

1. Strauss, Joseph. Green Book Commentaries, Volume XIV (2002), p. 17

CHIROPRACTIC LEXICON

GLOSSARY

In order to continue to explore the previously established central core of chiropractic, namely its principles and tenets, in a contemporary way we must rely on a base set terminology. As we move forward our educated intelligence grows and it requires that we progress without condemnation. The following glossary of terms was compiled, with the help of Joe Strauss, D.C., many of which are originally from Stephenson's text. Some additional terms that are uniquely needed for practicing the chiropractic objective have been incorporated.

100%/perfect: A quality of being free from all flaws or defect. It is the fullness of something material or immaterial.

Adaptability: (sign of life): The intrinsic ability that a living organism possesses to act on all information/force, which comes to it whether innate or universal.

Adaptation: The movement of a living organism or any of its parts, or the structural change in that organism, to use or to circumvent environmental information/force. Adaptation is a continuous process — continually varying, it is never constant and unvarying, as are other universal laws. Adaptation is a universal principle — the only one of its kind. It is the principle of change and the change is always according to law, which is 100%/perfect instantaneous integral adaptation.

ADIO (Acronym for Above-Down-Inside-Out):

1. An exclusive model of world viewpoint, under which chiropractic philosophy, logically and uncompromisingly, exists.

2. A thinking process with a unique perspective on life. First, there are absolutes in life (Prin. 1, 6, 20). Second, everything has a cause that should be addressed, if possible Prin. 17, 24). Third, there is a pre-eminence to the educated intelligence of humankind (Prin. 22, 27), a 100%/perfect universal intelligence (Prin. 1, 5).

3. Life comes from universal organization ABOVE (Prin 1,3), DOWN to living things' innate adaptation (Prin. 20, 23), expressing signs of life INSIDE the body (Prin. 18), to be manifested OUT as a living entity (Prin. 21).

4. In regards to coordination of activities of body parts (Prin. 32), in the vertebrate body, the innate impulse flows from the brain cell ABOVE (Prin. 28), DOWN to the tissue cell below (Prin. 18), is expressed from INSIDE the body part (Prin. 21), to be manifested OUT as coordinative purpose (Prin. 21, 32), according to universal laws (Prin. 24).

Adjustic thrust: An adjustic thrust is a specific, external, educated information/force introduced at the site of a subluxated vertebra with the intent that the innate law of living things will adapt to perform a vertebral adjustment.

Afferent nerve: The nerve that transmit trophic impulses from receptor tissue cell to central processing brain cell for coordination of activities. It is the route of feedback information/force from tissue cell to brain cell. It not to be confused with sensory nerves, which transmit sensory impulses from sense organs to physical brain.

Assimilation (sign of life): The ability of a living organism to selectively take food materials into its body and make them a part of itself according to a systematic program designed by a universal intelligence.

Characterization: The construction of specific codes by the universal principle of organization that organizes universal information/force in order to maintain energy/matter in existence; it is also the reconstruction (modified for living energy/matter) of specific codes by the innate law of living things that adapts universal information/force into innate information/force.

Chiropractic Meaning of Existence: It is the expression of the universal principle of organization through ALL energy/matter, living and non-living.

Chiropractor: One who knows the science, art and philosophy of Chiropractic and how to adjust subluxated vertebrae by placing in apposition the articular processes of the vertebral column.[2]

Chiropractor's vision: The chiropractor's vision is to insure the availability of chiropractic care to EVERYONE now and forever.

Chiropractic objective: The chiropractic objective is to locate, analyze, and facilitate the correction of vertebral subluxations for the normal transmission of the innate impulses of the body. PERIOD! The chiropractic objective is derived directly from the thirty-three principles of chiropractic's basic science.

Coding: The assignment of specific characters to identify a specific communication system programmed to construct a message.

Computation: The operation of a computing system. It is the processing of data of a computing system using a software program.

Counterfactuals: They are facts not about what is "actual" but about what is possible or not possible. For example, Dead Sea scrolls exist somewhere "hidden" on our planet. That is a physical property of those scrolls since they do exist. That it ***could be possible*** to read the words on them is a counterfactual property regardless of whether those scrolls would ever be discovered. And yet that those words ***could be*** read would still be true.

De-coding: To convert a coded message into intelligible language that can be understood.

Disease and DIS-EASE: Disease is a term used by physicians for sickness. To them it is an entity and is worthy of a name, hence diagnosis. DIS-EASE is a chiropractic term meaning not having ease; or lack of ease. It is lack of an entity. It is a condition of energy/matter when it does not have the property of ease. Ease is the entity, and DIS-EASE the lack of it.

E/matter: This term means energy-matter. Since $E=mc^2$, energy and matter are interchangeable; energy is simply a different configuration (properties) of electrons, protons, and neutrons with varying velocities (activities). For example, water has 2 molecules of hydrogen and 1 molecule of oxygen, whether it is in a fluid state, ice state, or vapor state. It is dependent upon the movement of its basic elements. It is a term reminding us that energy and matter are interchangeable as per $E=mc^2$, and that matter is comprised of electrons, protons, and neutrons configured at less than the square of the speed of light.

Educated brain: That part of the brain used by innate law of living things, as an organ, for reason, will, memory, education, and the voluntary functions.

---

2. Palmer, B.J., "The Science of Chiropractic, Its Principles and Philosophies." 4th Ed., Davenport, IA: The Palmer School of Chiropractic - Chiropractic Fountain Head. (1920) p. 12

Educated control: Educated control (also known as educated mind) is the activity of innate law of living things in the educated brain as an organ. The output of this activity is educated impulses such as thoughts, reasoning, will, memory, etc.... The innate law of living things controls the functions of the voluntary systems via the educated brain. Educated impulses are modified innate impulses that have passed through the educated brain and are mostly for adaptation to things external to the body.

Educated impulse: The innate information/force through the educated brain that becomes modified with whatever quality the educated mind can give it for the voluntary functions of the body. Note that the educated brain "controls" nothing, except that the innate information/force passes through it. Adaptation of information/force is ALWAYS and ONLY through the coding of innate impulses by the innate law. When innate impulses pass through the educated brain, they are "tinctured" and modified into educated impulses so there can be conscious action.

Educated Intelligence: The capability of the educated brain to function. It starts at 0% at birth and reaches its maximum limit at the death of the body (since it will develop no further).

Educated information/force: Educated information/force is innate information/force that has been modified by the educated mind for voluntary functions. It is really an educated impulse.

Efferent nerve: The transmitting nerve of innate impulses from the central processing brain cell to the receptor tissue cell. It is the route of conducted innate information/force from brain cell to tissue cell.

Energy: Electrons, protons, and neutrons configured at the square of the speed of light ($E=mc^2$).

E/matter: Energy/matter is electrons, protons, and neutrons configured at specific velocities in time.

Existence: The continuous motion of elemental particles of E/matter.

External educated information/force: An external educated information/force is innate information/force that has been voluntarily modified by the educated intelligence with a new educated character for so called voluntary action with a definite purpose. Ex: An adjustic thrust.

Flow: The action of something moving along in a steady continuous stream. In the body, it is the smooth continuous movement of information/F from one place to another.

Growth (sign of life): Growth is the ability of a living organism to expand according to intelligent programming to mature in size and is dependent upon the power of assimilation.

Hard to vary explanation: An explanation that provides specific details that fit together so tightly that it is impossible to change any detail without affecting its whole. In the case of chiropractic, the principles of its basic science are the hard to vary explanation of chiropractic.

Impression: It is the information/force coded by the innate law as trophic impulses, based on the complexity of the tissue cell concerning its soundness and functions.

Information/F: Information/force are computed and coded instructions to configure electrons, protons, neutrons, and their velocities.

Inforuns: Inforuns, (also known as foruns) are non-discrete information/force units that are continually organized by the universal principle of organization providing properties and actions to all E/matter in order to *maintain* it in existence (Prin.1, 8). Inforuns must be adapted by the innate law of living things and constructed into innate impulses for coordination of activities of all the parts of the body, or into innate rays/waves for cellular metabolism in order to *maintain* E/matter alive (Prin. 21, 23).

Innate control: Innate control (also known as innate mind) is the activity of the innate law in the innate field. It is the introduction of innate instructive information/F, as governance, into E/matter via the innate field of the body of **living** things to **maintain** the material of the body alive within the limits of adaptation (Prin. 21, 24).

Innate field: The innate field (also know as innate brain) is:
> a) That aspect of the living body used by the innate law of living things, as an operating system, in which to adapt universal information/F and assemble them,

> b) That facet of a living organism controlled by the innate law of living things, as an operating system, in which to assemble innate impulses, innate rays or innate waves, trophic impulses, and sensory impulses.

Innate impulse: Innate impulse (also known as mental impulse) is unit of information/F for a specific body part, for a specific function, for coordination of activities. A specific instruction given to a body part, for coordination of activities, for the present moment.

Innate information/F: Innate information/force (also known as innate force) is universal information/force adapted by the innate law of living things and codified for use in the body. It is assembled for dynamic functional process to cause tissue cells to function or to offer resistance to the environment. It is transmitted by nerve conduction from the brain to the tissue cell and is called an *innate impulse* when it impels parts of the body for coordinated action; it is called an *educated impulse* for voluntary actions; it is called a *trophic impulse* for feedback from the state and functions of body parts to the brain; when it is radiated from within all cells of the body for metabolism it is called an *innate ray/wave*; and it is called a *sensory impulse* when it is transmitted by sensory nerve from sense organs to the brain for adaptation to the environment. It is constructive toward structural E/matter (Prin. 26). Chiropractic ONLY addresses the innate impulse. Chiropractic does NOT address the educated impulse, the trophic impulse, the innate ray/wave.

Innate law of living things: The innate law of living (also known as innate intelligence) is the inborn organizing principle governing the body of a living thing through adaptation in order to **maintain** it alive, only if it is possible according to universal laws. It is the essential continuation of the universal principle of organization that is expressed through living E/matter keeping it alive through multiple levels of complex organization. It implements design, programming, self-correction, adjustability and adaptation to internal and external effectors.

Innate ray/wave: A unit of information/F for a specific tissue cell unit to keep it metabolically sound and alive for a specific unit of time within limitations of E/matter.

Instantaneous integral adaptation: Instantaneous integral adaptation (also known as intellectual adaptation) is the 100%/perfect cooperative processes of the innate law of living things to compute ways and means of adapting universal information/F and E/matter for use in the body and for coordination of activities. The interoperability of the innate law, in the innate field, to keep ALL the complexities of the living things organized to **maintain** it alive if it is possible according to universal laws (Prin. 21, 23, 24).

Instantiation: The act of producing a specific application of a principle. It is a process to deduce an individual statement from a general principle; the representation of an idea in the form of an instance of it.

Interoperability: A characteristic of the innate law in the innate field adapting information/F, the interface of which is completely understood to work with ALL the systems of the body, at present or in the future, moment to moment in either implementation or access.

Intra-cell particulates: Components of a cell adapted through innate information/F, in the form of innate rays/waves, that have been specifically coded by the innate law to process innate-normal metabolism (Prin. 27) for soundness of the cell.

Invasive information/F: Universal information/F acting powerfully upon tissue in spite of the innate resistance of the body, or in cases where the resistance of the body is lowered.

Matter: Electrons, protons, and neutrons configured at *less* that the square of the speed of light.

Mission of the chiropractic profession: The mission of the chiropractic profession is the specific task of increasing the awareness of the UNIVERSAL values of chiropractic for EVERYONE through education and by practicing the chiropractic objective.

Modifier: A slight change transforming a specific code through educated control that manifests innate impulses into educated impulses for voluntary functions.

Momentum: The possession of motion that is compounded by the mass of E/matter moved and its velocity. It is the active movement of E/matter in time. In chiropractic, momentum is the active frequencies of motion of the transmitting E/matter (neuron-transmitters) within the vertebrate body. Mass x Velocity = Momentum. Also momentum is subject to interference through being transferred from one element of information/F to another by vertebral subluxations. The *total* momentum of E/matter of the living body is always conserved.

Motor nerve: The nerve that transmits educated impulses (modified innate impulses) from the central processing brain cell to the receptor tissue cell. It is the route of educated functions from brain cell to tissue cell for voluntary actions.

Myo-vector: A chiropractic term describing the directional work of an operating para-vertebral muscle, adapted by the innate law, to process a vertebral adjustment for the correction of a vertebral subluxation within the limitations of E/matter (Prin. 23, 24, 31a, 31b). Utilized in ADIO analysis, a myo-vector reveals that the vertebra is not, at that moment, correctly positioned and interfering with the transmission of innate impulses.

Objective chiropractor (OC): An Objective Chiropractor is one WHO chooses to practice EXCLUSIVELY the chiropractic objective and nothing else.

Penetrative information/F: Invasive information/F that acts powerfully assailing the body and that has effect upon tissue in spite of the innate resistance of the body.

Physical brain: That part of the central nerve system used by the innate law of living things, as an organ, to centralize innate impulses that will be conducted across nerves for distribution to all the parts of the body for coordination of actions. It is also the organ of adaptation including the faculties of memory, will, and reason.

Poison: Any substance introduced into or manufactured within the living body, which the innate law of living things cannot process for metabolism.

Principle: A fundamental truth that is the foundation of universal laws.

Purpose of chiropractic: The purpose of chiropractic is to restore the momentum of transmission of innate impulses through the location, analysis and facilitation of the correction of vertebral subluxations.

Resistive information/F: Internal innate information/F that opposes invasive or penetrative information/F. It may manifests in many forms, physical, chemical, or mechanical. It is not called resistive information/F unless it is of that character. It is necessary for keeping ALL information/F in balance within the body.

Sensory nerve: The nerve that transmits sensory impulses from the perceptible tissue cell sensor to the brain cell processor. It is the route of special sense functions from the external impressions detected by a tissue cell sensor to a brain cell processor to adapt to the environment. Not to be confused with the afferent nerves used for feedback for coordination of activities.

Trophic impulse: Information/F that has been characterized by the innate law providing specific feedback information of the metabolic and coordinative state of a tissue cell. A trophic impulse is transmitted through afferent nerves from tissue cell to brain cell for coordination of activities. Not to be confused with the sensory nerves.

Universal information/F: Information/F organized **by** the universal principle of organization that is manifested by physical laws; it provides properties and actions to all E/matter that maintains it in existence; it is deconstructive toward structural E/matter (Prin. 26).

Universal intelligence: The fundamental CAUSE in chiropractic. Philosophically, it is the capability of the universal principle of organization to organize all of the infinite information/F, in the universal field to provide the properties and the actions of all E/matter **maintaining** it in existence (Prin. 1). It is the cause of organization due to the fact that organization bespeaks intelligence.

Universal principle of organization: The fundamental principle (major premise) of chiropractic's basic science intrinsic to all E/matter. The universal principle of organization is continually organizing all E/matter supplying properties and actions to all E/matter in order to maintain it in existence. It is the initial condition of chiropractic's basic science that organizes E/matter maintaining it in existence.

Vertebral adjustment and chiropractic adjustment: A vertebral adjustment is the correction of a vertebral subluxation caused by the process of adapting information/F by the innate law of living things. A chiropractic adjustment is the application of an adjustic thrust by a chiropractor, at the specific site of a vertebral subluxation, with the intent that the innate law will adapt this specific educated information/F to process a vertebral adjustment.

Viability: The capability of E/matter to live.

Vibration: The motion of a tissue cell performing its function.

Vitality: The soundness or integrity of a tissue cell. It is the quality of liveliness of a cell.

INTRODUCTION

ART. 1. REMARKS

The chiropractic knowledge contained within the pages of these volumes is written for the chiropractic student. It is new, re-contextualized work of the efforts that began in 1895. It acknowledges chiropractic's original roots and reinforces, what has been established by the discoverer, D.D. Palmer and the developer B.J. Palmer that chiropractic is unique, separate and distinct from everything else, and is inclusive of everyone. It also acknowledges that chiropractic facilitates the correction of vertebral subluxations, for a normal transmission of innate impulses conducted through the nerve system, which is the chiropractic objective. The chiropractic objective satisfies the principle of coordination. By restoring the transmission of innate impulses, chiropractic removes the cause that violates the principle of coordination. It also recognizes the axiom, "we cannot give what we do not have." If you have nothing to give, you can only give nothing.

ART. 2. CHIROPRACTIC DEFINED

1. "Chiropractic is a philosophy, science and art of things natural; a system of adjusting the segments of the spinal column by hand only, for the correction of the cause of DIS-EASE."[3]

2. "Chiropractic is the natural philosophy of life and health, and the art and science of properly locating, analyzing, and correcting vertebral subluxations in accordance with that philosophy."[4]

3. "Chiropractic is a philosophy, art, and science concerned with the restoration and maintenance of health."[5]

4. "Chiropractic is the philosophy, the science, and the art of specifically locating, analyzing and correcting vertebral subluxations in accordance with the principles of its basic science."[6]

The first definition is limiting chiropractic to adjusting "by hand only." The second definition is "in accordance with the philosophy," which is constantly growing, evolving, and being developed, thus bound to change. The third definition is "concerned with the restoration and maintenance of health," which happens only sometimes, and is limited to a fraction of the human experience, namely health.

The last definition is by far the most appropriate for the re-contextualization of chiropractic in the 2020s. It states exactly what chiropractic is with simplicity and precision. It is based on the absolute testability and verifiability of the immutability of most principles of chiropractic's basic science. It is thus a definition of chiropractic that is hard to vary. This chiropractic definition concludes that chiropractic is unique and that the chiropractic objective is based on the accurate and precise principles of chiropractic's basic science. It delineates, with crystal clear certainty, the practice of chiropractic, the application of these established principles for the restoration of transmission of innate impulses through the correction of vertebral subluxations. The chiropractic objective is achieved every time a specific chiropractic pre-check is performed and the interference with transmission of innate impulses has been removed by the

---

3. Stephenson, R.W. "Chiropratic Text Book" (Vol. XIV) Davenport, IA: The Palmer School of Chiropractic (1948) p. xiii

4. Gold, Reginald. Sherman College Course Philosophy 801 Notes, Spartanburg, SC (1976) p. 5

5. Gelardi, Thom. "Sherman College of Chiropractic 76-78 Catalog" Spartanburg, SC: Sherman College of Chiropractic (1976) p.12

6. Lessard, Claude. "Timed Out: Chiropractic." Self-published, Claude Lessard D.C. (2022)

innate law of living things (through the correction of vertebral subluxation) and verified with a specific chiropractic post-check. The momentum transmission of innate impulses, from input to output, is thus restored within the limitations of E/matter. It also includes the three aspects of chiropractic, nothing more, nothing less, nothing else.

Throughout the text, the student will be given ample opportunities to verify or falsify the accuracy of this re-contextualized definition of chiropractic.

ART. 3. SCIENCE, ART AND PHILOSOPHY

Those three aspects are taken for granted in current debates within the chiropractic curriculum. A variety of techniques have been developed over the decades. It is clear that the art portion of chiropractic has evolved over the last century in terms of analysis and adjusting techniques. The understanding of the philosophy has evolved from a therapeutic model (getting sick people well) toward a non-therapeutic model (location, analysis, and correction of vertebral subluxations to restore the normal transmission of innate impulses exclusively). The third component of chiropractic, science, had been less well defined and developed until, in 2017, when *A New Look At Chiropractic's Basic Science* was published. The 33 principles were shown to be not philosophical concepts but testable and verifiable scientific principles. The 33 principles were then reclassified within the foundational body of the basic science component of chiropractic. In 2022, another book was published titled, *Timed Out: Chiropractic,* where it demonstrated and further clarified that chiropractic's basic science is definitely the unifying link between the philosophy and the art. The principles of chiropractic's basic science become a "*G*uiding *P*rinciple *S*ystem" (GPS) to keep the chiropractor on course, in order to exclusively practice the chiropractic objective, through error corrections, what B.J. Palmer called, "checking our slippings."

Chiropractic philosophy provides an explanation of chiropractic that is hard to vary, based on the principles of chiropractic's basic science. Since we cannot give what we do not have, we can use those principles by analogy. We can construct data processing computers that are a copy of the human body, which is truly a super data processing computer, that includes a 100% perfect innate software. Human beings use their bodies the same way they use various devices to move their intentions from one place to another. For example, cell phones and laptops to communicate with other people, homes to shelter ourselves, automobiles to move from one town to another, airplanes to move from one continent to another and so on. All information transportation is subject to code (signal) interference that can cause a change of momentum and coherence in transmission, thereby altering communications. Every mode of communication in use is an intellectual or physical expression of the human being and must be kept free from interference in order to function the way it was intended. It is the responsibility of human beings to maintain their devices free from code signal interference to best express themselves, and that includes their bodies as data processing super computers. Regarding the device called the human body, an interference called the vertebral subluxation violates the principle of coordination of actions. Of course we must always keep in mind that the human body belongs to the Animal Kingdom, and that we are much more than animals. The human body, as a biological data processing device, belongs to the Theory of Systems Organization, and we must remember that we are much more than computers. This clarification will be fully developed during this course of study as we explore the educated intelligence of the human brain.

The definition of chiropractic states that it is "the philosophy, the science and the art of properly locating, analyzing and correcting vertebral subluxation in accordance with the principles of its basic science." This simply means WHAT chiropractic is, HOW chiropractic is applied and practiced, and WHY. Science tells us WHAT it is. Art tells us HOW it is practiced. Philosophy tells us WHY chiropractic does what it does and how it does it. Accordingly, it is the science that informs the philosophy. The immutable principles of chiropractic's basic science direct the explanation of chiropractic that is hard to vary and unite it to the art including its conclusive practice objective.

ART. 4. SCIENCE

There is an aspect of chiropractic, central to the understanding of chiropractic that has so far been neglected. It is the science aspect of chiropractic. It is partly due to having classified the 33 chiropractic principles under the aspect of chiropractic philosophy. They were thought to have been philosophical concepts, while in fact those principles of chiropractic are scientifically testable and verifiable. They are factual and they can be used to predict the correction of vertebral subluxations, if it is possible, within the limitations of E/matter.

The Merriam-Webster Dictionary defines *science* as:

> **1:** The state of knowing: knowledge as distinguished from ignorance or misunderstanding.

> **2:** A department of systematized knowledge as an object of study.

> **3:** Knowledge or a system of knowledge covering general truths or the operation of general laws especially as obtained and tested through scientific method.

> **4:** A system or method reconciling practical ends with scientific laws.

Chiropractic's basic science is comprised of 33 principles that can be applied to locate, analyze, and facilitate the correction of vertebral subluxations (see Art. 23). Those principles are testable and verifiable, and ultimately dictate the chiropractic objective with accuracy. The chiropractic principles comprise "a system of knowledge covering general truths." They belong to "a department of systematized knowledge as an object of study." The principles of chiropractic's basic science become "a system or method reconciling practical ends with scientific laws." This will be thoroughly demonstrated throughout this work with the current knowledge of the 2020s. This work will also identify the link between chiropractic philosophy and the art of chiropractic as being the principles of chiropractic's basic science.

ART. 5. ART

The Merriam-Webster Dictionary defines *art* as:

> **1:** Skill acquired by experience, study, or observation.

> **2:** A branch of learning: one of the humanities.

> **3:** An occupation requiring knowledge or skill.

> **4:** The conscious skill of creative imagination.

The art of chiropractic consists of skills in analysis and adjusting techniques most requiring hours of study, learning and practice. It also includes communication skills. The art of communicating the chiropractic objective, and the location, analysis and facilitation of the correction of vertebral subluxations is based upon "the conscious use of skill and creative imagination" that the chiropractor has developed over time from classroom studies, internship within chiropractic facilities, and externship programs.

ART. 6. PHILOSOPHY

The Merriam-Webster Dictionary defines *philosophy* as:

1a: All learning exclusive of technical precepts and practical arts.

1b: A discipline comprising as its core logic, aesthetics, ethics, metaphysics, and epistemology.

2a: Pursuit of wisdom.

2b: A search for a general understanding of values and reality by chiefly speculative rather than observational means.

2c: An analysis of the grounds of and concepts expressing fundamental beliefs.

3a: A system of philosophical concepts.

3b: A theory underlying or regarding a sphere of activity or thought

4: The most basic beliefs, concepts, and attitudes of an individual or group

Literally philosophy is the love of wisdom. It is in the narrowest sense, nearly equivalent to metaphysics. It is "an analysis of the grounds of and concepts of expressing fundamental beliefs."

In more general application, philosophy denotes a "discipline comprising at its core, logic, aesthetics, ethics, metaphysics, and epistemology… a system body of philosophical concepts," ordinarily with the implication of their practical application.

ART. 7. CHIROPRACTIC PHILOSOPHY

Chiropractic philosophy is "a system of philosophical concepts (and/or a theory) regarding a sphere of activity and thought" that gives an explanation of why chiropractic exists. Simply put, it answers "why" chiropractic does what it does and how it does it. It concerns itself with all the studies of chiropractic based on its basic science and applied science. Chiropractic philosophy suggests explanations that are hard to vary and transmits its body of knowledge for the benefit of all. Chiropractic philosophy is the torchbearer where the chiropractic flame is passed on from one to the other to ignite the world afire. The starting point of chiropractic philosophy, as we will see later in the text, is the innate law of living things that maintains the body alive, as long as it is possible without breaking a universal law. Chiropractic philosophy concerns itself with the activity and thought of living systems.

ART. 8. CHIROPRACTIC IS A DEDUCTIVE SCIENCE

Chiropractic is a radical science comprised of a universal principle that explains scientific laws used to construct a solid platform, the bedrock upon which chiropractic can rest. It aims to restore the transmission of conducted innate information/F. It removes interference to the transmitters of innate impulses to satisfy the principle of coordination. Chiropractic is a radical science in so far as it does not concern itself with effects; chiropractic is only about cause! The starting point of chiropractic's basic science is its fundamental principle (major premise) that is assumed from scientifically verified observations. This original principle is an a priori statement. It is the initial condition of chiropractic's basic science. From Principle 1, we apply deductive reasoning to formulate a cascade of subsequent minor principles, axioms, that eventually reveal the chiropractic objective, which is the ending point of chiropractic. Chiropractic is a human necessity that includes everyone without exceptions.

Chiropractic is a deductive science. The deductions are based upon an initial principle that the entire universe is organized. This principle is called the universal principle of organization. It is derived from observations and has been verified as being a universal truth. From chiropractic philosophy, we acknowledge and understand that organization bespeaks intelligence. The universal principle of organization was designed, constructed and programmed by a universal intelligence so that all of E/matter is maintained in existence. Therefore, the deductions are further based upon an initial condition that existence is organized and intelligent!

There are seven characteristics of chiropractic's basic science:

> 1. Chiropractic is unique and vitally important for everyone regardless of their personal values or beliefs systems.
>
> 2. Chiropractic consists of a systematically organized body of knowledge that forms its basic science (33 principles). Most of the principles are immutable and have for conclusion an absolute irrefutable objective.
>
> 3. Chiropractic is an experimental method that applies the 33 principles to the practice the chiropractic objective.
>
> 4. Chiropractic is reproducible in facilitating the correction of vertebral subluxations.
>
> 5. Chiropractic principles are verifyable through the chiropractic objective.
>
> 6. Chiropractic makes specific predictions from its basic science to achieve the chiropractic objective through its applied science.
>
> 7. Chiropractic is focused on natural things, ie cells, organs, functional systems, and living vertebrate bodies.

The theories and hypotheses of chiropractic are based upon proven deductions from the initial fundamental principle of its basic science. These will be further developed and will be the key subjects of these four volumes.

To maintain all E/matter in existence through a universal principle of organization that provides all of its properties and actions is awe-inspiring! Especially as we consider that it is possible for E/matter to have multiple levels of structural organization that increases in complexity toward living and thinking E/matter. The universal trajectory moves from condensed E/matter to more and more complex and highly organized states of E/matter, all the way to manifesting signs of life, namely living E/matter. This organizing principle is further designed, developed, constructed, and programmed by a universal intelligence into an innate law of living things. The function of the innate law is to adapt universal information/F and living E/matter, for use in the body to maintain it alive for a period of a lifetime, without breaking a universal law.

Note to the student: No matter how awe inspiring, it is important not to characterize and endow this universal intelligence with divinity. Divinity belongs to the study of theology. Deism and theism are not chiropractic. Chiropractic is a philosophy, a science, and an art! Chiropractic is not a religion. This universal intelligence did not and does not create energy, matter, or information out of nothing. This universal intelligence designed, developed, and programmed a universal principle that organizes every bit of reality that already existed to maintain it in existence. With regard to living E/matter, this universal intelligence further modified, designed, and programmed this universal principle into the innate law of living things that adapts universal information/F and E/matter for use in the body. Creation, the big bang, natural selection, evolution, mysticism, ontology, anthropomorphism, deism, theism, divinity, spirituality, religion, the occult, and God are all outside and beyond the realm of chiropractic philosophy, science, and art. It is the reason why, as we mentioned already, chiropractic is available to everyone regardless of their personal values or beliefs systems.

ART. 9. TERMINOLOGY-LEXICON

Chiropractic is separate and distinct from everything else. Chiropractic has its own terminology and a unique lexicon that serves to communicate its philosophy, science, and art. It is important that the lexicon of chiropractic clarifies the exact meanings for the intents and applications of the principles of its basic science. Any conversation about its philosophy, science, or art requires an agreement of terms to transmit and disseminate the hard to vary explanation of chiropractic. This vocabulary is provided throughout the text and can be referenced in the glossary.

ART. 10. INDUCTIVE REASONING

Inductive logic is a type of reasoning that draws a general conclusion from a set of specific observations. By definition, inductive reasoning, or induction, is making an inference based on an observation, often a sample. It is a movement from the specific to the general, from the part to the whole. It is the logic of the reasoning of empirical science. It is a posteriori, which means inductive, compared to a-priori, which means deductive. Inductive reasoning is more of a synthesis. "It reasons that the whole thing is like any of its parts, the conclusion being based upon a representative number of parts, going from the specific to the general."[7] Inductive reasoning is, at times, used in chiropractic through observations. For example in Art. 8, we assumed teleologically, through observation, that organization bespeaks intelligence. We explain the existence of a universal intelligence through its function instead of its cause. Hence we can state that a universal intelligence does exist, that it designed, developed, constructed, and programmed the universal principle of organization to maintain every bit of E/matter in existence. This assumptive induction is the initial condition that comprises the fundamental principle as the starting point of chiropractic's basic science.

---

7. Stephenson, "Chiropractic Text Book" p. xviii

REVIEW QUESTIONS ARTICLES 2-10

1. Give the definition of chiropractic used for this re-contextualized textbook.

2. Why is it the best definition for 2022?

3. Why is chiropractic not limited to human beings only?

4. What is the art of chiropractic?

5. What is chiropractic's basic science?

6. What is chiropractic's applied science?

7. What is chiropractic philosophy?

8. Why is the chiropractic definition in accordance to the principles of its basic science?

9. What is the initial basis of chiropractic?

10. Why is chiropractic a radical science?

11. What is the starting point and the ending point of chiropractic?

12. What is inductive reasoning?

13. Why is deductive reasoning best suited for chiropractic?

14. Why is it important not to endow intelligence with divine characteristics?

15. Why does chiropractic need its own lexicon?

ART. 11. LABORATORY

The Merriam-Webster Dictionary defines *laboratory* as:

1a: A place equipped for experimental study in a science or for testing and analysis; a place providing opportunity for experimentation, observation, or practice in a field of study.

1b: A place for testing, experimentation, or practice.

According to Stephenson's research, Webster stated in 1927 that a laboratory was… "A place devoted to experimental study in any branch of natural science, or the application of scientific principles in testing and analysis…" Laboratory is suitable for inductive reasoning as parts are observed to construct the whole. Observations may yield to prove or disprove certain principles. Chiropractic uses laboratory observations, at times, as we will encounter during our study of some of the chiropractic principles. Inasmuch as chiropractic does not use inductive reasoning often, some conclusions reached to verify certain principles are based on a synthesis of observations that are then reasoned through deductive reasoning as we further study chiropractic. Laboratory findings present facts that are often useful to verify certain chiropractic principles. Chiropractic can be constructed on a solid a priori foundational bedrock platform as long as the initial condition of an assumptive principle is based on reason and scientific verification. Some facts gained from laboratory work can then be applied to verify or falsify chiropractic principles.

ART. 12. DEDUCTION

The Merriam-Webster Dictionary defines *deduction* as:

1a: An act of taking away.

1b: Something that is or may be subtracted.

2a: The deriving of a conclusion by reasoning; an inference in which the conclusion about particulars follows necessarily from general or universal premise.

2b: A conclusion reached by logical deduction.

Chiropractic assumes an initial condition in the form of a fundamental universal principle that organizes every bit of E/matter in order to maintain it in existence. This initial assumption has been scientifically proven through laboratory experiments, that a universal principle of organization governs all E/matter. Organization bespeaks intelligence. Organization is one of the functions of intelligence. The initial assumption is that the maintaining of existence is intelligent. Every particular thought derived from that initial principle, that is thoroughly analyzed, is verifiable, if and only if, the fundamental principle is true. If the fundamental principle is true and the deductive reasoning is sound, then the conclusion will be true and will become the final condition. Deductive reasoning, is also referred to as above-down thinking. At its most basic deductive reasoning is to draw conclusions from a general true principle using rational logic. For example, "Every individual is mortal. D.D. Palmer is an individual. Therefore D.D. Palmer is mortal." In chiropractic, deductive reasoning is the method used rationally and logically to conclude its objective.

This raises the question, "Can deductive reasoning be false?" Deductive reasoning can lead to a false conclusion if one of the premises is false. As a general principle, whenever one supposes that something is true and then reaches a contradiction, one can conclude that the assumption is false. For example, if one assumes that "Only chiropractic gets sick people well and a sick person got well today, one would conclude that this person must be under chiropractic care." In this example, the conclusion would be true if the two premises were true. However, the original assumption that "*Only* chiropractic gets sick people well" is not true. In fact, chiropractic never heals anyone of anything. Only the body's self-healing system heals. Therefore the conclusion is also not true. If the principles from which the conclusion is derived are true, then the conclusion must also be true.

Its counterpart is inductive reasoning, often referred to as below-up thinking. It draws conclusions based on premises that are not automatically true but are believed to be. For example, if it is believed that "Every chiropractor practicing the chiropractic objective went to Sherman College, then it can be concluded that only chiropractors who went to Sherman College practice the chiropractic objective." The assumption is not true and therefore the conclusion is not true.

Inductive reasoning is often not true, even if the original premises are true. For example, "Chiropractic sometimes gets sick people well" is true. "A sick person got well today," is true. Therefore, that person must be under chiropractic care. In this example, both premises are true yet the conclusion is not necessarily true. Just because chiropractic sometimes gets sick people well does not mean that every sick person getting well is under chiropractic care. It does not necessarily correlate that this sick person who got well today was under chiropractic care.

Through deduction of an incorrect premise, such as "the earth is flat," an erroneous conclusion can be derived, "one might eventually reach the end of the earth." However, when the erroneous conclusion is not verified by evidence, the initial assumption must be questioned for validity. This is how "Chiropractic gets sick people well" was asserted by chiropractors for many years until Reggie Gold, D.C. saw the opportunity to make an error correction by clarifying "sometimes." He further tested this hypothesis, and today we understand that chiropractic is only about the restoration of transmission of conducted innate information/F, and this happens "all the time" when vertebral subluxations are corrected. It is the chiropractic objective, which is the conclusion of the 33 principles of chiropractic's basic science, and it is based on deductive reasoning and rational logic. Reggie's reasoning refuted the "chiropractic gets sick people well" theory, and as a result established that chiropractic is non-therapeutic. This revision illustrates how deductive reasoning, in chiropractic, is essential for of error correction, and therefore for the progress of chiropractic as a whole. When rational logic as a whole proves deductions to be wrong they automatically become problematic and are usually dismissed in favor of alternative ones.

Induction can also be a means for arriving at conclusions. Many hypotheses are based on assumptions and analyzing conclusions drawn from these assumptions can lead to new discoveries. For example, D.D. Palmer concluded that he had found the cure for deafness from what he had observed and assumed in 1895. That was a wrong assumption. Further testing, from D.D. himself, allowed him to discover that "to replace displaced vertebrae by using the spinous and transverse processes as lever into their normal position… to restore all morbific conditions."[8] From this new discovery, D.D. Palmer constructed a science that was destined to revolutionize all human activities.

---

8. Palmer, B.J. and D.D. Palmer. "The Chiropractic Adjuster." Davenport, IA: The Palmer School of Chiropractic (1921) p. 316

ART. 13. CLINIC

The Merriam-Webster Dictionary defines *clinic* as:

> **1:** A class of instructions in which patients are examined and discussed

> **2:** A group meeting devoted to the analysis and solution of concrete problems or to the acquiring of specific skills or knowledge

> **3a:** A facility of health care for outpatients

> **3b:** A facility that offers professional services or consultation usually at discounted rates

Clinical, by way of definition, possesses all the contrasts of thought and introduces the opposite. Clinic is where immaterialism enters everything materialistic, where the very process of reasoning is admitted to be the method of procedure in elucidation.[9] Clinic, in chiropractic, is where non-discrete dictates everything discrete. It is really a private session where the spinal analysis of the practice member is conducted. It is where communication and the actual relationship between practice member and chiropractor is established. It incorporates the factual knowledge of the organizing principle that governs the living E/matter of the subject in question and thus is thus clinical. The chiropractor corrects the interference to transmission between brain cell and tissue cell, (between E/matter and E/matter) that causes a lack of ease of the neuron-transmitters altering the momentum of transmission of innate impulses. When this interference is corrected, which restores the transmission of innate impulses it normalizes the computation process of the organizing principle which is intrinsic to living E/matter to manifest motion (Prin. 14, 15). The expression of living E/matter is then innate-normal (Prin. 13, 27). The meaning of clinic in chiropractic is the recognition of the governance of a non-discrete organizing principle, which is intrinsic in all discrete living E/matter.

The contrast between laboratory and clinic is that a laboratory is where facts are drawn from scientific experiments and a clinic is where the chiropractor and subject encounter a specific human experience at a certain moment in time. Clinical experience is not a laboratory and it is not scientific. Clinical experience deals with the subject with its physical, mental, emotional, and abstract components. It is where deductive reasoning takes places and can be applied, in the clinical setting, which includes the principles of chiropractic's basic science, their assumptions, and a priori statement. Clinic is where chiropractic's basic science merges into applied science to put its principles into practice through the art of chiropractic.

ART. 14. AXIOMS

The Merriam-Webster Dictionary defines *axioms* as:

> **1:** A statement accepted as true as the basis for argument or infererence

> **2:** An established rule or principle or a self-evident truth: for example,
> *cite the axiom that "no one gives what he does not have"*

> **3:** A maxim widely accepted on its intrinsic merit

Chiropractic works with the application of the established principles of its basic sciences. These axioms are the solid bedrock on which chiropractic is constructed. It is not clear today if truths are definable at

---

9. Stephenson, "Chiropractic Text Book" p. xxi

all. They seem to be related to the properties and actions given by an organizing principle intrinsic to all E/matter that mainbtains it in existence. For example, organization bespeaks intelligence is an axiom that proves the existence of intelligence based on its function and not its cause. It is a statement accepted as true as the basis of a teleological argument. It is accepted without controversy or question. A universal principle is used to construct universal laws; it includes a hard to vary philosophical explanation.

One needs first to have two rival theories concerning a physical situation to which the principle purports to apply. For example, one can consider organization being the consequence of randomized possibilities versus organization being the consequence of intelligent certainties. Then one performs an experiment with an actual system of organization to test the prediction of one model against the other. This will be demonstrated later on in the text as we study the initial condition of chiropractic's basic science, a universal principle of organization.

When we look at the nature of the chiropractic model, we see it as the embodiment of a set of axioms that have cascaded through deductive reasoning and rational logic, from its major premise. The initial condition of chiropractic's basic science is its fundamental principle, which is its major premise. From this starting point of chiropractic's basic science, rational logic and sound deductive reasoning are used to formulate axioms that will conclude in and reveal the chiropractic objective. The initial condition of an organizing principle is an irreducible primary. It doesn't rest upon anything to be valid and cannot be proven by other principles. It cannot be invalidated because any attempt to do so can only end in a contradiction. In other words, it cannot be denied without using it in our denial. However, the universal principle of organization can be observed, as we will also demonstrate later in the text.

ART. 15. PARADOXES AND PARADIGMS

The Merriam-Webster Dictionary defines *paradox* as:

> **1:** One (such as a person, situation, or action) having seemingly contradictory qualities or phases
>
> **2a:** A statement that is seemingly contradictory or opposed to common sense and yet is perhaps true
>
> **2b:** A self-contradictory statement that at first seems true
>
> **2c:** An argument that apparently derives self-contradictory conclusions by valid deduction from acceptable premises
>
> **3:** A tenet contrary to received opinion

Paradoxes have been part of the human experience for as long as the human race has existed. Paradoxes have value in chiropractic philosophy because they provide an awareness of ways to look at the human body that are logically convincing with seemingly legitimate convincing arguments that lead to a conclusion which is contradictory.

For example, chiropractic colleges and universities find it necessary to teach from the medical model, as truth, to their students so that they won't be disadvantaged in the "real" world. By doing so, these institutions negate the validity of chiropractic's basic science, its philosophy, and practice. One cannot ascribe to two diametrically opposed philosophies at the same time; it is a "self-contradictory conclusion."

Most chiropractic students are not aware of this philosophical conflict, yet the opposing models they are taught are programmed into the formation of their chiropractic minds. No wonder most chiropractic graduates of the 2020s have had their confidence undermined to such an extent as to choose the conventional medical "accepted approach" of practice, which is "to get sick people well." This is an academic paradox within chiropractic. Paradox simply comes from a limited point of view. The paradox often results from thinking *inside* the box as opposed to thinking *outside* the box. The student should "see" what is to be seen with a different set of eyes. Often paradoxes will reveal a new way to look at the subject of study. Chiropractic is a new look at the human body. One that reveals a universal intelligence that has designed, constructed, and programmed a universal organizing principle and its essential extension, the innate law of living things. For this reason, it is necessary to introduce the term paradigm in order to proceed with our subject study.

The Merriam-Webster Dictionary defines *paradigm* as:

> **1:** EXAMPLE, PATTERN *especially*: an outstandingly clear or typical example or archetype
>
> **2:** An example of a conjugation or declension showing a word in all its inflectional forms
>
> **3:** A philosophical and theoretical framework of a scientific school or discipline within which theories, laws, and generalizations and the experiments performed in support of them are formulated: a philosophical or theoretical framework of any kind

A paradigm is a blueprint that contains all the commonly accepted views about a subject. Philosopher Thomas Kuhn suggested that a paradigm includes "the practices that define a scientific discipline at a certain point in time."[10] For example, a chiropractic paradigm consists of all the established principles and axioms comprising chiropractic's basic science, including its philosophy and practice, that allow us to recognize an objective as belonging to chiropractic or not.

Many students who choose to study chiropractic do so with the belief that they are receiving an education based on the most rational path to learning its philosophy, science, and art. But chiropractic, like other disciplines, is subject to ideological utopias, preconceptions, and hidden assumptions.

In 1927, the chiropractic textbook conditioned and shaped the interpretations that the chiropractic objective was to get sick people well. The certainty that this 1927 paradigm was the real objective of chiropractors is precisely what makes it so difficult to accept a different objective.

Kuhn wrote, "The successive transition from one paradigm to another via revolution is the usual developmental pattern of mature science."[11]

For over 100 years, chiropractors were convinced that "getting sick people well" was the pinnacle of discovery in chiropractic and that progress was more or less a refinement of its procedures to achieve this more effectively. When Reggie Gold published "The Third Paradigm" in the 1990s, which will be included completely in Volume 4, it was a new idea that did not fit comfortably into the existing paradigm. It pointed out a truth, namely that chiropractic gets people well only sometimes. It led to a crisis. The previous paradigm was challenged and brought about a new order of reclassification of the principles of chiropractic's basic science, as we saw in Art. 3. It is an essential in the 2020s, as the paradigm shifts! Chiropractic is being developed further. It does not completely disprove the old paradigm. It merely points to the fact that chiropractic get sick people well only sometimes and that the

---

10. Kuhn, Thomas S. "The Structure of Scientific Revolution." Chicago, IL: The University of Chicago Press. (1962)

11. Kuhn, "The Structure of Scientific Revolution." p.12

33 principles of chiropractic's basic science dictate that, the chiropractic objective is to locate, analyze, and facilitate the correction of vertebral subluxations for a normal transmission of the innate impulses of the body. Period. The chiropractic objective is the direct conclusion from the deductive reasoning and rational logic of the 33 principles of its basic science; the chiropractic objective is more precise, delivers more powerful predictions, offers fruitful research programs and is more consistent than what it was previously thought to be. Now when the principles are applied through practice, the chiropractic objective is achieved all the time and not just sometimes. It can be verified from pre and post checks.

Chiropractic is not developed in a linear way, gradually accumulating knowledge and deepening its explanations. Rather, it alternates between periods of practice within a dominant paradigm and periods of revolutionary shifts when an emerging crisis requires a NEW paradigm. It becomes as defined *a philosophical and theoretical framework of a scientific school or discipline* called chiropractic's basic science, within which its theories, generalizations, principles and axioms are formulated and applied in practice. As we will later develop in the text, that is what this new paradigm means in chiropractic philosophy.

ART. 16. THEORIES AND FACTS

Chiropractic's basic science is "WHAT" chiropractic consists of. It is comprised of established facts that are derived from principles and axioms. It has theories as how to best apply those principles and axioms that are deduced thereof for the practice aspect of chiropractic. Those theories are the philosophical explanations of the facts. They are not random guesses or personal opinions. Theories are time-tested explanations for why we observe "HOW" chiropractic does "WHAT" it does and "WHY." A theory can be discarded for a better one or can be re-constructed at different times due to new knowledge that has been discovered.

The Merriam-Webster dictionary defines *theory* as:

> **1:** Explain phenomena
>
> **2a:** A belief, policy, or procedure proposed or followed as the basis of action
>
> **2b:** An ideal or hypothetical set of facts, principles, or circumstances
>
> **3a:** A hypothesis assumed for the sake of argument or investigation
>
> **3b:** An unproved assumption: CONJECTURE
>
> **3c:** A body of theorems presenting a concise systematic view of a subject
>
> **4:** The general or abstract principles of a body of fact, a science, or an art
>
> **5:** Abstract thought: SPECULATION
>
> **6:** The analysis of a set of facts in their relation to one another

Theories are our best explanations for why all the observations are happening. Much more than a solution to a particular problem, they are conjectured explanations that attempt to approximate principles and laws of the universe, the rules that constrain everything in our universe. Theories are words to explain the core content that the chiropractic principles express. Without philosophy a principle is empty and has no meaning. Without principles, the philosophical explanation, the theory is too vague to be applied. The two conditions are indissoluble. A chiropractic theory, therefore is not just the set of its principles, such as the universal principle organization or its essential extension which is the innate law of living things, it is an explanation that is hard to vary, which includes descriptions of what existence and life are in principles, and why they are related in that way. For example, why can water change from liquid to solid, back to liquid, and then can change to vapor? Why are energy, matter, and information never created or destroyed? Why for every action is there an opposite reaction? The answers to these questions are explanations that are hard to vary, that we also use in chiropractic. They are directly related to the universal principle of organization that continually maintains in existence all of the elemental particles of E/matter through organized information/F providing continuous motion (Prin. 1, 13, 14, 15). It is an explanation that is hard to vary; it is a theory that is hard to vary! Since the universal principle of organization approach is hard to vary, it is natural to wonder whether it could have the power to be extended to explain everything about the universe itself. In other words, would the initial condition of chiropractic's basic science, which is the universal principle of organization be able to provide a satisfactory explanation for every bit of reality in the universe? The answer, as you are about to discover, in this text, is no. The universal principle of organization of chiropractic's basic science is an excellent initial condition for maintaining all E/matter in existence. However, it cannot explain everything about physical reality. In fact, when regarded as an explanation of everything, the organizing principle has serious problems. That is why we need chiropractic philosophy to explain universal organization as bespeaking a universal intelligence, which is non-discrete, non-material, and 100%/perfect. A universal intelligence that has designed, constructed, and programmed the universal principle of organization and the innate law of living things to provide properties and actions to all E/matter. It should be noted though that the universal principle of organization and the innate law of living things are excellent explanations for specific purposes; a universal principle of organization to maintain E/matter in existence, and the innate law of living things to maintains E/matter alive for a lifetime.

A universal theory is one that is not subject to any limitation regarding its domain of applicability. Chiropractic's initial condition is a fundamental principle of its basic science, its major premise, and it maintains in existence every bit of E/matter on Earth, within the solar system, in fact, within the entire universe. It is as defined *an ideal set of facts, principles; it is the general principles of a body of fact, a science, or an art.*

The Merriam-Webster Dictionary defines *fact* as:

> **1a:** Something that has actual existence
>
> **1b:** An actual occurrence
>
> **2:** A piece of information presented as having objective reality
>
> **3:** The quality of being actual
>
> **4:** A thing done

Facts are the result of scientific inquiry. From a philosophy standpoint, facts stand or fall on the strength of the disciplines and practices that produced them and made them understandable rather than on the strength of their own truth. When we seek facts, we are attempting to discover what is true about an event or an object. Therefore, it is true that facts are dependent on theories that are explanations for their existence. Hence, our view of the facts "changes" as the theories that imply them change. Since we simply cannot collect ALL the facts, it is very difficult to state anything with utmost certainty about any given situation, even if our initial presumption is that we should leave no stone unturned. We may be able to collect as many facts as we can and still not have them all. Therefore, in order to move forward in chiropractic, we must select only the most relevant and important facts to build upon. This selection is one of the amazing characteristics of the chiropractic deductive process. When chiropractic's basic science has for its initial condition a fundamental a priori statement saying that there is a universal principle of organization, the deduction of the other axioms, like the innate law of living things, become fact as much as the existence of the organizing principle itself given that our logic is properly applied. It is as defined *something that has actual existence, the quality of being actual.*

ART. 17. EXAMPLES

The Merriam-Webster Dictionary defines *example* as:

> **1:** One that serves as a pattern to be imitated or not to be imitated

> **2:** A punishment inflicted on someone as a warning to others

> **3:** One that is representative of all of a group or type

> **4:** A parallel or closely similar case especially when serving as a precedent or model

> **5:** An instance (such as a problem to be solved) serving to illustrate a rule or precept or to act as an exercise in the application of a rule

An example is used to illustrate its point. It is an instance to act as an exercise in the application of a rule, a principle or axiom.

ART. 18. ANALOGIES

The Merriam-Webster Dictionary defines *analogy* as:

> **1a:** A comparison of two otherwise unlike things based on resemblance of a particular aspect

> **1b:** Resemblance in some particulars between things otherwise unlike

> **2:** Inference that if two or more things agree with one another in some respects they will probably agree in others

> **3:** Correspondence between the members of pairs or sets of linguistic forms that serves as a basis for the creation of another form

An analogy is a comparison that demonstrates how two different entities are similar, showing a most important point due their common relationships. Analogies are a way of comparing entities that helps to clarify them. It often constructs images for the student to understand the deeper concepts of chiropractic. It can enhance the meaning of concepts.

Examples and analogies will be used throughout the text to clarify the principles and axioms involved in chiropractic. They are a parallel of closely similar cases. The examples and analogies are not the actuality in question, simply a representative, an instance that demonstrates the way a principle works. It is drawing a comparison to show similarity in some respect, like the operation of a super computer presents a great analogy in 2022 to the workings of the whole body. The examples show by analogy how the body is programmed with a 100%/perfect software, using an operating system in coordinating all its parts. This is not to convey that the human body is a computer, but that it belongs to the computer systems classification the same way that it belongs to the animal kingdom. It is the relationships that are being compared, not their personal natures. Sometimes the analogy breaks down as we delve into it. The computer analogy is good up to a point. When the non-material component enters the picture in the form of 100%/perfect software, the analogy breaks down. The human body is more than a computer due to the 100%/perfect innate law that never needs updates, and it is more than animals due to our educated intelligence and volition. The analogy is helpful, yet it has limits. The reason we can construct computers is because we can copy some of the properties and actions of the already existing body of living things using its principles. As we work backward from computers we can use them as an analogy to explain the inner workings of the human body. We can program software that includes operating systems, and we can construct hardware, CPU, data processors, and transmitters, due to the fact that we are able to copy some principles that are inter-acting in human body. The analogy of the universal computer generated a new chiropractic principle called, "The principle of continuous supply and computation." The principle of continuous supply and computation is existent in the body in its ideal state; wherein the living body is the "computer," the innate law is the "normal software," the innate field is the "operating system," the brain is the "central processing unit," the brain cells are the "processors," and the nerve cells are the "transmitters." (Prin. 33)

ART. 19. THE THREE PHASES OF CHIROPRACTIC STUDY

1. Study of the non-material (non-discrete)

2. Study of the material (discrete)

3. Study of the art

The study of the non-material, which is non-physical (non-discrete), involves examining the fundamental nature of reality through philosophy. It includes the study of intelligence, principles, laws, causes, effects, theories, functions, etc. It is about understanding existence and knowledge. It is to discover or construct knowledge from the principles of chiropractic's basic science. Non-material means not to have physical form. While the instructive message of the information/F carried by the innate impulse is non-material, it must be conducted through the material nerve system of the body.

The study of the material, which is physical (discrete), is the study of substances and components that make up a thing. It is the study of E/matter and of the principles of chiropractic's basic science that are central to it; it is also the study of the human body, its elemental units, its structures and its functions. It is the study of universal facts. Given that chiropractic is the study of existence and the study of life, learning of the E/matter that makes up the human body fosters a greater understanding of chiropractic as a whole, especially for the student who has a good knowledge of universal laws regarding E/matter.

When studying academic courses regarding the human body, the student should look for "WHY" the body is "WHAT" it is, and "WHY" it works "HOW" it works its intelligent functions, as well as, the significance of its integrated structural forms. There should always be an awe struck reason as to what is being observed, studied and learned regarding the amazing wisdom continually manifested by the body, that is, "HOW" it acts, and "WHY" it acts the way it does.

The study of art is learning the very practical nature of chiropractic as it applies to locating, analyzing, and correcting vertebral subluxations. It is the chiropractor's attempt to understand, describe, and facilitate the vertebral adjustment. In truth, it is the application of the principles of chiropractic's basic science as an art form. It requires the development of skills and takes practice in order to be an effective chiropractor; the same way that a musician practices long hours to develop the skills to play an instrument very well. The study of the art is learning "HOW" to restore transmission of conducted information/F necessary for the body to satisfy the principle of coordination. It is about, with specific expertise, deconstructing patterns of interference to the conducted instructions of the innate law that further increase the limits of adaptation of the body. In other words, it is to bring about what is not possible with the presence of vertebral subluxations to what is possible without vertebral subluxations.

The three phases of chiropractic study include non-physical essentials, such as intelligence, universal principle of organization, innate law of living things, and some of their deduced axioms. Chiropractic is a vitalistic approach to every facet of human life. Chiropractic entails what is possible for the body without vertebral subluxations, with its known facts and also its essential counterfactuals (see definition in lexicon).

In the long range perspective, the development of chiropractic will require the progressive understanding and implementation of the principles that govern its ability to restore the link between the non-material and the material, between the non-discrete organizing principle and the discrete E/matter, by removing the interference called vertebral subluxation.

ART. 20. A COMPARISON

Sitting on a dock of the bay in Ocean City, New Jersey during early evening twilight, in August, an amazing spectacle happens. As the sky darkens, many different kinds of lights and sounds arise. The bay becomes enchanted with signaling lights coming from boats moving across the water, with music from the shore's bars, with the green beacon from the small airport that flashes on and off.

All these systems have something in common. The boats' lights, the music, and the airport beacon, they are all signals. They are carrying information; they can link entities together. Boats' lights link boaters to avoid collisions with each other. The music links musician and audience bringing a delightful mood. The airport beacon links airplanes for traffic control. The fact that they can, in fact, code messages to connect entities is extremely important to understand existence and life. Information is the link that connects the non-material with the material; it is at the heart of everything. This discovery could further revolutionize our civilization, such as removing interference to this information-link within the human body. The innate impulse is also capable of carrying a coded message through the conductivity of the nerve system.

This fact reveals the chiropractic objective, which is to restore the link between intelligent/principle and energy/matter. The chiropractic objective is not attempting to improve the intelligent/principle that is 100% perfect. It is not to improve E/matter per se, since we do not know how it should be. It is to remove interference at the vertebral level that will restore the transmission of conducted information/F. It aims to restore the momentum of the innate impulse because timing is most important for all activities (Prin. 6).

For example, to perform a symphony, to bake a cake, to teach a course, or to play hockey, all of theses activities require proper timing to be most effective. The activities of the human body are also subject to the momentum of coded innate impulses, for better or for worse.

Chiropractic is about the link between discrete and non-discrete, its area of interest. As we will point out later in the text, without this understanding, the student may stray away from the link in either or both directions, either by attempting to improve intelligence/principle or by attempting to improve energy/matter.

ART. 21. THE MISSING LINK

The striking singularity of chiropractic science, both basic and applied, is that it is based upon the link between non-discrete intelligent/principle and discrete energy/matter. These four volumes will explain in great details this actual link. It is the activity of information/F that is intrinsic to every single manifestation of motion of E/matter. It is this activity that maintains every particle of E/matter in existence; it is from the universal principle of organization, which is the initial condition of chiropractic's basic science, its fundamental principle, its major premise, that information/F is organized in such a way as to provide properties and actions to all E/matter. It is called the "missing link" as it was not recognized until chiropractic discovered that information/F was the bond (strong and weak) between the non-material and the material.

Well over one hundred years later, the missing link has been on the cusp of a pernicious boundary that would exclude the connection between the non-discrete and the discrete. It seems that the traditional conception was that everything that happens in the universe could be explained through mechanistic processes that involve only physical laws. This has created a barrier against the non-physical factor of reality, and if taken literally, is impossible. First of all, it is not possible to explain everything in terms of physical laws. We would have to know all of them and the universe is too voluminous for that. Even if it were possible, we would soon realize that there has to be a universal organizing principle causing these physical laws intrinsic to E/matter that are constructed to maintain everything in the universe in existence. Universal organization bespeaks a universal intelligence and it has a non-discrete property. For example, in data processing, why is a given transmitter of a certain computer "ON" at the end of a certain computation, has many possible answers? Which one is the real answer? It is essential for the software to have been programmed to know the "real" answer every time a computer performs a certain function. This organization of computation was engineered and programmed by a non-material aspect of reality (the engineer's knowledge) that constructed the appropriate software.

Organization bespeaks intelligence. It is impossible to have organization without intelligence. For example, the highly complex construction of a computer is comprised of some already existing universal elements that have been organized by computer engineers. It would be impossible for you to assume that this extremely complex computing system would be organized without a non-discrete intelligence. Chiropractic is about what is possible. So, the universal principle of organization has been designed and constructed by a non-discrete universal intelligence to organize information/F, to maintain in existence every particle of discrete E/matter in the universe. This philosophical explanation is hard to vary. Both non-material and material aspects of reality are united through the continual intelligent organization of information/F intrinsic to all E/matter. It is the missing link! This is a universal fact that chiropractic alone has discovered. This a-priori statement is the initial condition of chiropractic upon which D.D. Palmer constructed a science, an art, and a philosophy that is a humanitarian revolutionary approach to life. It is his son, B.J. Palmer, who then further developed the chiropractic philosophy, science, and art.

Chiropractic philosophy is therefore the hard to vary explanation of the working principles of its basic science. It is also the explanation of everything chiropractic, the non-material, the material, and the art of its practice. Chiropractic philosophy is not spirituality, or mysticism, or ontology, or occultism. Chiropractic addresses the interference in momentum of the transmission of conducted information/F. It is the area of expertise that chiropractors develop their skills to apply the principles of chiropractic's basic science. This is the chiropractors' unique approach, not to attempt to affect E/matter, not to attempt to affect the intelligent organizing principle, but to focus attention on the missing link, that which unites the intelligent organizing principle to E/matter (See Prin. 10).

REVIEW QUESTIONS ARTICLES 11 - 21

1. What is the main reason why chiropractors sometimes use laboratory findings?

2. What is deductive reasoning?

3. What is the main characteristic of deductive reasoning?

4. What is another term for deductive reasoning?

5. What is the meaning of clinic in chiropractic?

6. What is clinical experience and why is it not scientific?

7. What is an axiom?

8. Why is chiropractic so simple fundamentally?

9. What is a paradox?

10. What is a paradigm?

11. What is a fact?

12. What is a theory?

13. What aspect of chiropractic deals with theory?

14. What is the origin of the first chiropractic theory?

15. How were the chiropractic facts obtained?

16. What is an example?

17. What is an analogy?

18. What are the three phases of chiropractic?

19. What is "THE MISSING LINK?"

20. What is the value of the principles of chiropractic's basic science?

21. What is the chiropractor's unique approach?

22. What is non-discrete and bespeaks intelligence?

ART. 22. PRINCIPLES

The Merriam-Webster Dictionary defines *principle* as:

1a: A comprehensive and fundamental law, doctrine, or assumption

1b: A rule or code of conduct

2a: The laws or facts of nature underlying the working of an artificial device

2b: A primary source: ORIGIN

Principles are general rules that govern disciplines such as chiropractic, biology, laws of physics. An example is Newton's three laws of motion or Einstein's formula ($E=mc^2$) and so on. In physics, the uncertainty principle is described as "nothing has a definite position, a definite trajectory, or a definite momentum." In chiropractic, the organizing principle is a fundamental principle, which is described as "the organization of information/force to supply properties and action to every bit of E/matter, thus maintaining it in existence (Prin. 1). As define within our lexicon, a *universal principle is a fundamental truth that is the foundation of universal laws.* The principles of a science are its governing laws, which may be comprehensive and fundamental instructions of its operation. Any activity of the human body has guiding instructions to provide rules of operation regarding those activities.

For example, aviation has its principles of aerodynamics of how air moves around objects, comprised of the forces of lift, drag, weight, thrust, and so on. These forces make an aircraft move up and down, faster or slower. Flight has sequence, harmony, balance, variation, phases, all which are rules governed by the principles of aerodynamics. Chiropractic has its organizing principle and laws called the universal principle of organization and the innate law of living things that demonstrate how every bit of E/matter is maintained in existence through organized motion and how it can, at times, be maintained alive for a lifespan through its adaptability according to its limitations. Those principles are fundamental to chiropractic and they bespeak intelligence. Principles are important in life, and the 33 principles of chiropractic science are the foundational guiding instructions for the study and the practice of chiropractic.

ART. 23. THE PRINCIPLES OF CHIROPRACTIC'S BASIC SCIENCE

Chiropractic's area of study is life in all its grandeur. It concerns, more specifically, vertebrate animal bodies. However, its initial principle is a fundamental condition that concerns the existence of every bit of E/matter in the universe. It is the universal principle of organization; organization bespeaks intelligence; the processes or actions of the universal principle of organization are intelligent and are always maintaining E/matter in existence. This fundamental principle includes any and all circumstances that may arise in study.

We will be studying 33 principles that have been selected to construct chiropractic's basic science. They are not the only principles of chiropractic, just 33 that have been chosen because they are deduced fundamentals for the student to understand chiropractic as a humanitarian evolutionary approach to life.

ART. 24. A LIST OF THIRTY-THREE PRINCIPLES OF CHIROPRACTIC'S BASIC SCIENCE NUMBERED, NAMED, AND RE-CONTEXTUALIZED[12]

UNIVERSAL PRINCIPLES

No. 1. The Major Premise
A universal principle of organization is continually supplying properties and action to all energy/matter, thus maintaining it in existence.

No. 2. The Chiropractic Meaning of Existence
The expression of this organizing principle through energy/matter is the chiropractic meaning of existence.

No. 3. The Union of the Principle of Organization and E/matter
Existence is necessarily the union of the universal principle of organization and energy/matter.

No. 4. The Triune of Existence
Existence is a triunity having three necessary united factors, namely, the principle of organization, information/force and energy/matter.

No. 5. The Perfection of the Triune
In order to have existence, there must be 100%/perfect organizing principle, 100%/perfect information/force and 100%/perfect energy/matter.

No. 6. The Principle of Time
All processes require time and space.

No. 7. The Perfection of the Organizing Principle in Energy/Matter
The perfection of the organizing principle for any particle of energy/matter is always 100%/perfect and complete.

No. 8. The Function of the Principle of Organization
The function of the principle of organization is to organize information/force.

No. 9. The Amount of Information/Force
The information/force organized by the principle of organization is always 100%/perfect.

No. 10. The Function of Information/Force
The function of information/force is to unite the principle of organization and energy/matter.

No. 11. The Character of Universal Information/Force
The information/force of the universal principle of organization is manifested by physical laws; is unswerving and unadapted, and has no solicitude for the structures in which it works.

No. 12. Interference with Universal information/force
There can be interference with the transmission of universal information/force.

No. 13. The Function of Energy/matter
The function of energy/matter is to express information/force.

---

12. Lessard, "Timed Out: Chiropractic." p. 144-148

No. 14. Existence

Information/force is manifested by motion in all energy/matter; all energy/matter has motion, therefore all energy/matter has existence.

No. 15. No Motion without Instructive Information/Force

Energy/matter can have no motion without instructive information/force supplied by the principle of organization.

No. 16. Organization in both Organic and Inorganic Energy/Matter

The principle of organization governs both organic and inorganic energy/matter.

No. 17. Cause and Effect

Every effect has a cause and every cause has effects.

No. 18. Evidence of Life

The signs of life are evidence of the adaptive organization of life.

No. 19. Organic Energy/Matter

The material of the body of a living thing is organic energy/matter.

INNATE PRINCIPLES

No. 20. Innate Law of Living Things

A living thing has an inborn organizing principle governing its body, called the innate law of living things.

No. 21. The Purpose of the Innate Law of Living Things

The purpose of the innate law of living things is to maintain the material of the body of a living thing alive.

No. 22. The Quality of the Innate Law of Living Things

The innate law of living things is always 100%/perfect for all living energy/matter.

No. 23. The Function of the Innate Law of Living Things

The function of the innate law of living things is to adapt universal information/force and energy/matter for use in the body, so that all parts of the body will have coordinated action for mutual benefit.

No. 24. The Limits of Adaptation

The innate law of living things adapts information/force for the body and energy/matter only if it is possible according to universal laws.

No. 25. The Character of Innate Information/Force

The information/force of the innate law of living things never injures or deconstructs the structures in which it works.

No. 26. Comparison of Universal Information/Force and Innate Information/Force

In order to carry on the universal cycle of life, universal information/force is deconstructive, and innate information/force is reconstructive, regarding structural energy/matter.

No. 27. The Normality of the Innate Law of Living Things

The innate law of living things is always normal and its function is always normal.

No. 28. The Conductors of Innate Information/Force
The conducted information/force of the innate law of living things operates through or over the nervous system in animal bodies.

No. 29. Interference with Transmission of Conducted Innate Information/Force
There can be interference with the transmission of conducted innate information/force.

CHIROPRACTIC PRINCIPLES

No. 30. The Cause of DIS-EASE
Interference with transmission of conducted innate information/force causes incoordination of DIS-EASE.

No. 31. The Vertebral Subluxation and its Correction
    a. The vertebral subluxation is the uniquely chiropractic entity as a cause of interference to the transmission of conducted innate information/force,

    b. and the correction of a vertebral subluxation is always due to the process of adapting information/force by the innate law of living things.

No. 32. The Principle of Coordination
Coordination is the principle of coherent actions of all the parts of an organism in fulfilling their roles and purposes.

No. 33. The Principle of Continuous Supply and Computation
The principle of continuous supply and computation is existent in the body in its ideal state wherein the living body is the "computer," the innate law is the "normal software," the innate field is the "operating system," the brain is the "central processing unit," the brain cells are the "processors", and the nerve cells are the "transmitters."

The 33 principles of chiropractic's basic science conclude with crystal clarity the exclusive chiropractic objective.

The Chiropractic Objective
The chiropractic objective is to locate, analyze, and facilitate the correction of vertebral subluxation for a normal transmission of the conducted innate information/force of the body. Period.

These 33 principles will be used for the concluding work of Volume One of the text. They are discussed in detail in Volume Four, but it is advisable to learn their names for reference at this point.

REVIEW QUESTIONS ARTICLES 22 - 24

1. What is the nature of a principle for a specific science?

2. What is a fundamental principle?

3. What are deduced principles and what is their purpose?

4. How many principles of chiropractic's basic science are used for our study?

5. What is a fundamental principle of chiropractic?

6. Could every particle of E/matter be maintained in existence without the universal principle of organization?

7. What does organization bespeak?

8. What are the three elements of existence revealed by chiropractic's principles?

9. What is required for existence to be maintained?

10. What is the quality of the innate law of living things?

11. What is the function of the innate law of living things?

12. What is the character of universal information/F?

13. Can universal information/F be interfered with?

14. What is the function of E/matter?

15. What is the evidence of the existence of E/matter?

16. What is the evidence of the existence of information/F?

17. Can an effect be without a cause?

18. What is the innate law of living things?

19. What are the signs of life?

20. What is organic E/matter?

21. What is purpose of the innate law of living things?

22. What is the difference between the organic E/matter of the wood of a tree and the organic E/matter of the wood of a chair?

23. What is the function of the innate law of living things?

24. Is the innate law of living things different in a bee than in a whale?

25. What determines if the adaptability of the body is possible?

26. What is the character of innate information/F?

27. Is the innate law of living things always normal?

28. What system of the body is used to transmit conducted innate information/F?

29. Why can there be interference with transmission of conducted information/F?

30. What does the interference with transmission of conducted information/F cause?

31. What is the cause of the interference with transmission of conducted information/F?

32. Where do we always find the cause of in-coordination of action in the body?

33. How does chiropractic deal with cause and not effects?

VOLUME 1

"This first of four Volumes…" "What Stephenson refers to as Freshman Text…" is the foundational work of chiropractic study. It includes the consideration of the principles and fundamentals, and is principally the careful examination of the Normal Complete Cycle. The student should undertake this task progressively throughout Volume One as concepts and ideas build upon each other.

ART. 25. CHIROPRACTIC

Chiropractic's basic science identifies a universal principle of organization that maintains everything in the universe as its initial and fundamental condition. This is manifested by motion and is called existence. A distinct and essential process of this organizing principle keeps alive a specific portion of E/matter, for a lifetime, and is called the innate law of living things. The function of an inborn innate law is to adapt some of the information/F and E/matter of the universe into individualized instructions to maintain a thing alive for a lifetime according to universal laws. (Prin. 23, 24)

Organization of living things points to centralization or point of control for coordination of activities. In animals, this center of control is the physical brain. The innate law governs and operates every living cell of a particular animal or organism. In vertebrate bodies, the innate law uses the brain in order to centralize and transmit its control via conducted information/F across the spinal cord through the spinal column. From there, it continues through the nerve trunks that emit from the spinal cord and pass through the inter-vertebral foramina to the nerve branches reaching to all parts of the body for coordination of activities.

Perfect adaptation from the innate law, for coordination of activities, depends upon the possible adaptability of the universal elements of that particular body. Perfect adaptation, for coordination of activities, requires complete control if it is possible (without breaking a universal law) and will satisfy the principle of coordination. Interference with that control will bring about a lack of ease and it will violate the principle of coordination.

Lack of ease is never due to any imperfection of the innate law, which is 100%/perfect and adapts 100%/perfect information/F, but from interference with the transmission of those conducted innate information/F through or over the nerves for coordination of activities. Since the spinal column is the only segmented structure of bone through which the nerve trunks pass, and since those segments can displace changing the size and shape of the inter-vertebral foramina, it is possible for vertebral subluxations to occur there. If vertebral subluxation occurs, it will cause an interference with the transmission of conducted innate information/F. Lack of ease of transmission causes loss of momentum of conducted innate information/F and will cause in-coordination of activities. Chiropractic is a science which consists of having scientific knowledge regarding this cause of lack of ease of specific neurons which alter the momentum of the transmission of the conducted innate information/F. It also includes the artistic ability to apply a specific adjustic thrust to facilitate the correction of a vertebral subluxation, thereby removing interference with the transmission of conducted innate information/F. The vertebral adjustment, which is computed and processed by the innate law, does not add or subtract any material to the body but simply allows the restoration of normal transmission that would have been had there been no interference. In this manner, the principle of coordination is fulfilled and satisfied.

Chiropractic includes the study of living things, but that of the vertebrate in particular and more specifically that of the living human body. At the present time adjustic thrusts are almost entirely confined to the human spine and the spines of a few domestic animal species to bring about coordination of actions of all the parts of that living body. Therefore, our studies, with the exception of the fundamentals, will be mainly related to:

1. The innate law of living things and its function regarding the coordination of activities the living human body and its connected parts

2. The proficiency that is required to facilitate the correction of the cause of DIS-EASE.

ART. 26. THE CHIROPRACTIC DEFINITION OF VERTEBRAL SUBLUXATION (SEE PRIN. 31)

A vertebral subluxation is the condition of a vertebra that has lost its proper juxtaposition with the one above or the one below, or both; to an extent less than a luxation; which impinges nerves and interferes with the transmission of innate impulses.

All of the factors of the foregoing definition must be included to accurately describe what a vertebral subluxation is and to make it a chiropractic explanation; nothing more, nothing less, nothing else. The student is advised to learn it word for word.

Dislocations, fractures, swelling of soft tissues, poisons, and other things, can also interfere with transmission of innate impulses, however they are outside the realm of chiropractic.

ART. 27. THE CENTRALIZATION OF CONDUCTED INNATE INFORMATION/F FOR COORDINATION OF ACTIVITIES

The innate law adapts universal information/F, encodes and assembles it into innate information/F and then must centralize the ones that will be conducted for coordination of activities. Centralizing is necessary to supply and process innate impulses, including feedback, regarding activities of all the receptor parts of the body. The organ used for centralizing the conducted innate information/F is the physical brain, the Central Processing Unit (CPU). From there the innate impulses will be transmitted through or over the nerves for coordination of all the parts of the body. The student is reminded that as an abstract, non-material principle, the innate law is intrinsic to every tissue cell of the body and is therefore everywhere in the body. It is only the innate impulses that are centralized for the coordination of activities of the parts of the body. Regarding metabolism of the tissue cell, the innate law encodes information/F into specific innate rays/waves that are then radiated/oscillated from within the tissue cell itself. It will be discussed later in the text as we study the innate information/F in depth. Both normal conducted and radiated/oscillated innate information/F converge for use in the body and for coordination of action of all its parts (Prin. 23). However, the practice of chiropractic concerns itself only with the conducted information/F, the innate impulse, as per the principles of chiropractic's basic science.

ART. 28. TRANSMISSION OF CONDUCTED INNATE INFORMATION/F FOR COORDINATION OF ACTIVITIES

The innate law centralizes the conducted innate information/F within the physical brain (CPU) then transmits them through the efferent nerves (transmitters) to be received by the parts of the body (receptors) for coordination of action.

ART. 29. EFFERENT NERVES (SEE PRIN. 28)

Efferent nerves are the nerves used for transmission of conducted information/F (innate impulses) from the physical brain to the receptor part of the body for coordination of activities. The word efferent indicates direction. According to the Merriam-Webster Dictionary, *efferent* is defined as: "conveying nervous impulses to an effector." This word is derived from Latin, effere, which means to carry outward. The route is from brain cell to tissue cell, from CPU to receptor.

Efferent nerves are transmitters of innate impulses and begin in the physical brain leading out through the spinal cord and emitting to all the parts of the body. Coordination of action of body parts would not be possible without such nerve supply.

ART. 30. AFFERENT NERVES (SEE PRIN. 28)

Afferent nerves are the nerves used for transmission of conducted information/F (trophic impulses) from the receptor part of the body to the physical brain, conveying feedback for coordination of activities. The word afferent also indicates direction. According to the Merriam-Webster Dictionary, *afferent* is defined as: "conveying impulses toward the central nervous system." This word is derived from Latin, affere, which means to carry inward.

Afferent nerves are transmitters of trophic impulses that originate in a part of the body and lead to the physical brain to provide feedback for coordination of activities. Coordination of action of body parts would not be possible without such nerve feedback. Philosophically, feedback must always be true to be a valid feedback whether normal functions or abnormal functions. Therefore, vertebral subluxations cannot interfere with transmission of feedback. This is corroborated and verified anatomically as vertebral subluxations cannot impinge upon afferent nerves since they run outside the spinal cord. Only efferent nerves can by impinged by vertebral subluxations (see following diagram).

Afferent Neurons
- Carry sensory info from Receptors in Skin/ other organs➔Central Nervous System
- Cell bodies are located OUTSIDE of the Spinal Cord

Autonomic Division
- Regulates involuntary body responses

Skin

Dorsal Root

Cell Body

Dorsal Root Ganglion

Blood Vessels

Skeletal Muscles

Spinal Cord Cell Body

Ventral Root

Efferent Neurons
- Carry motor info from Brains➔Peripheral Nervous System
- Cell bodies are located INSIDE of the Ventral Horn of the Spinal Cord

Somatic Division
- Voluntary movement by Skeletal Muscles

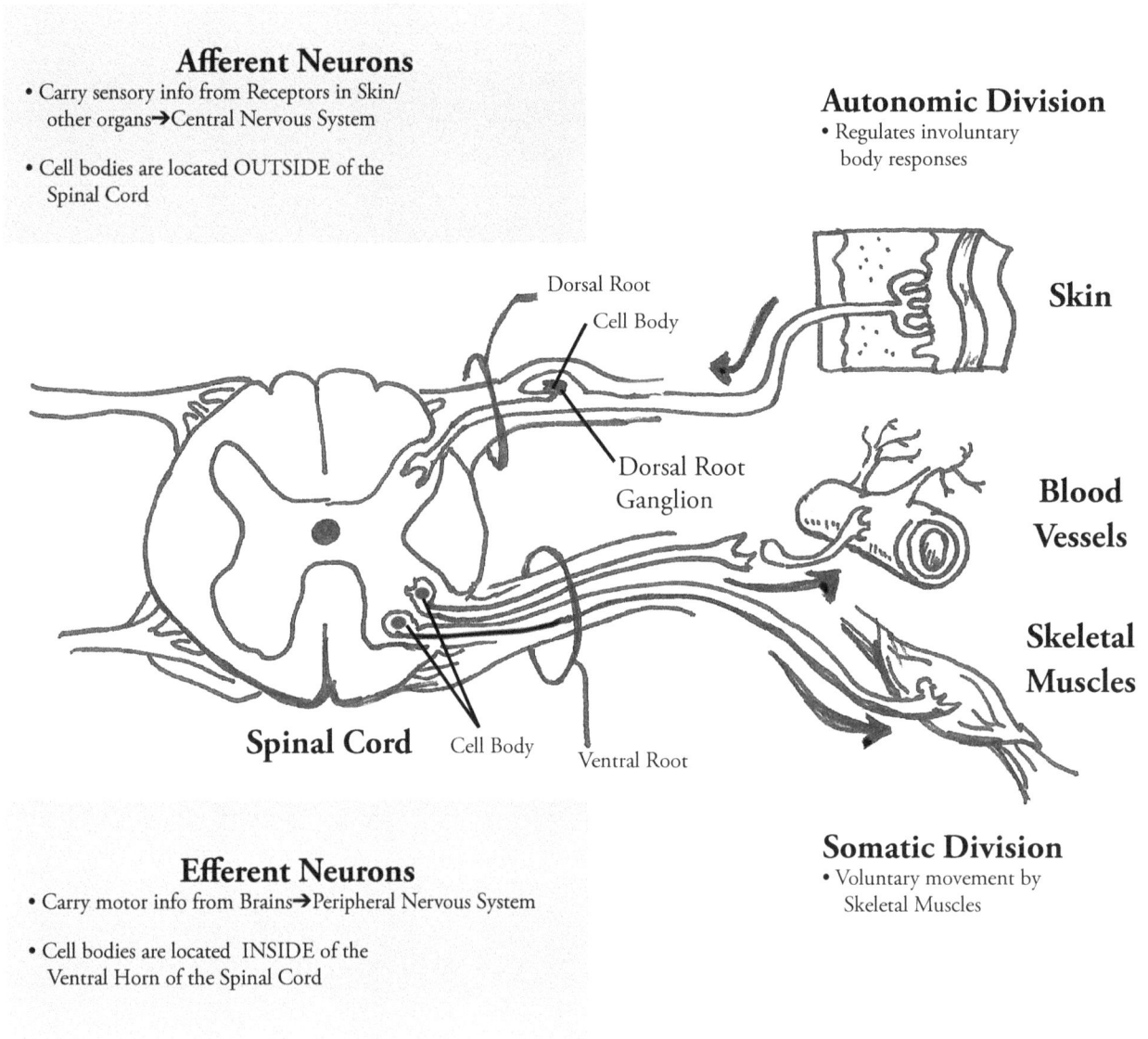

Fig. 1. Diagram demonstrating efferent nerves where the cell bodies are located INSIDE the ventral horn of the spinal cord and subject to impingement by vertebral subluxations and afferent nerves where the cell bodies are located OUTSIDE of the spinal cord and are NOT subject to impingement by vertebral subluxation.

ART. 31. THE NERVE CYCLE FOR COORDINATION OF ACTION (SEE PRIN. 28)

The innate law governs and operates the entire body including the physical brain, as CPU, to communicate with every part of the body for coordination of activities, by means of efferent nerves as transmitters, which extend from it. All the parts of the body have nerves for coordination of activities.

Similarly, the innate law governs and operates the parts of the body to communicate feedback to the physical brain by means of afferent nerves, which are connected to it. All parts of the body participate in this feedback loop system for coordination of activities.

Thus, there is a continuous supply of conducted innate information/F and feedback from the cycle of physical brain to physical body part that is continually being transmitted by the innate law through this pathway to fulfill the principle of coordination. It is a reciprocal relation between actual interoperability of biophysical systems governed and controlled by the innate law.

The dictum, "We cannot give what we do not have" is true in so far as we cannot construct that which cannot be copied. The principle must first exist so it can be discovered and applied for practical purposes. For example, computer engineers were able to construct computers because of the already existence of computation principles discovered from quantum mechanics, and from the law of continuous supply and computation that processes the biological data within the human body (Prin. 33). When we observe closely with the knowledge of the 2020s, the body is truly a supercomputer. When the innate law adapts universal information/F and E/matter, it is really computing and encoding them into innate information/F. Therefore, the act of adapting is basically the computating of information/F and the motion of E/matter, to maintain it alive for a lifetime according to universal laws (Prin. 23, 24). The human body belongs to the order of animal kingdom and to the theory of systems organization. Of course, we know that we are more than animals and we also know that we are more than computers.

The body is comprised of many cycles, such as the digestive cycle, the respiratory cycle, the circulatory cycle, the serous cycle, etc. For example, the circulatory system is a cycle between the heart and the blood vessels and the related tissues. Blood is pumped out of the heart through the arteries and returns to the heart through the veins. The purpose of the blood vessels is to carry the material things whether supplied or wasted that are coursing through them. The nerves, like the blood vessels, also carry something, however, what is carried by the nerves cannot be seen, for it is intangible. We can only perceive its effects or lack thereof.

This something, carried by the nerves, is conducted innate information/F (innate impulse) from the innate law for coordination of activities. The innate impulse is computed and coded as an instructive message by the innate law for coordination of action of all the parts of the body (Prin. 23). In 1927, the original chiropractic textbook used the term mental impulse to describe innate information/F. However, according to the Merriam-Webster Dictionary, *mental* refers to intellectual activity of the mind. The term mental is anthropomorphic. The more accurate term to describe the conducted innate information/F is innate impulse, which refers specifically to the activity of the innate law within the innate field. The innate law continually computes, encodes and assembles innate information/F. It is a 100%/perfect software continuously processing biological data moment to moment, the function of which is to adapt information/F and E/matter (Prin. 23). It then centralizes the innate impulses for coordination of activities of body parts, in the physical brain (CPU) so that they will be transmitted through the efferent nerves (transmitters) to be received by the intended body part (receptor). Then, the innate law uses the innate field of the receiving body part (receptor) to decode the innate impulse into impressions. At this point the innate law recodes these impressions into trophic impulses to provide feedback that is transmitted through the afferent nerves (transmitters) back to the physical brain (CPU). This is called the nerve cycle. The innate law continually computes, encodes, and recodes impulses to be transmitted as efferent supply and as afferent feedback to complete the nerve cycle for coordination of activities. The nerve cycle process continues over and over and over again for mutual benefit of all the parts of the body (Prin. 23) as long as it is possible according to universal laws (Prin. 24).

REVIEW QUESTIONS ARTICLES 25 – 31

1. Construct a simple description of chiropractic based on Art. 25.

2. Provide the chiropractic definition of vertebral subluxation word for word.

3. Explain why if any part of the definition would be missing it would not be a vertebral subluxation.

4. Can dislocations, fractures, and swelling of tissues interfere with the transmission of innate impulses? What should a chiropractor do about those?

5. What part of the body is the CPU?

6. What part of the body is the transmitter?

7. What part of the body is the receptor?

8. What is the function of an efferent nerve?

9. What is the function of an afferent nerve?

10. What is the "something" that both efferent and afferent nerves carry?

11. When does the nerve cycle cease to function in the living body?

ART. 32. INNATE INFORMATION/FORCE

Innate information/F is data, transmitted, conducted or radiated/oscillated, which unites the non-discrete organizing principle with the discrete living E/matter to maintain it alive, for a lifetime.

Conducted innate information/F is called innate impulse because it impels the body part to manifest coordination of activities which is an intelligent action. Radiated/oscillated innate information/F is called innate ray/waves because it maintains the tissue cell alive through radiation from within the tissue cell for its metabolism. All innate information/F eventually converges for use in the body and coordination of body parts for mutual benefit (Prin. 23).

Conducted innate information/F is an instructive message that is carried by nerves which are living E/matter. Remember that nerves are conductors of innate impulses in animal bodies for coordination of activities (Prin. 28). All innate information/F, from the innate law, is necessary to control and balance everything in the body to maintain it alive according to universal laws (Prin. 23, 24).

Innate information/F is non-material until it unites the organizing principle with E/matter. At that specific moment, innate information/F is both non-material and material. That is why innate information/F is called innate impulse. It refers to the fact that it is information reorganized into a non-material instructive coded message to be conducted as an impulse, a coded message conveyed through or over material (chemo-electric) E/matter as conductor. Basically, the transportation system is the organized motion of electrons, protons and neutrons of the nerve cells that give rise to the momentum of the coded message transmission. The encoded instructive message is the characterization of universal information/F into innate information/F through the function of the innate law. The actual union is the instant where the non-material and material interface with each other in the body for coordination of activities. This will be studied in depth later in the text.

As previously stated, there can be interference with the transmission of universal information/F (Prin. 12). Therefore, since the innate law of living things is an essential extension of the universal principle of organization, it follows that there can be interference with the transmission of innate information/F (Prin. 29). As an example, putting up an umbrella to cast over a patch of a flower garden will interfere with the universal information/F of sunrays and rain. If a nerve is impinged there will be a lack of ease of that particular nerve that will interfere with the transmission of the innate impulse and change its momentum. This in turn will violate the principle of coordination (Prin. 33). Chiropractic is concerned with the restoration of the transmission of the innate impulse. Of course, if the nerve is severed, the transmission of the innate impulse ceases completely and the body part will not receive any instructive message at all. The condition and organization of the integrity of the body are dependent upon the governance and control of all its parts by the innate law.

ART. 33. LOCATION OF THE INNATE LAW IN ORGANISMS

The non-discrete innate law is intrinsic to every discrete tissue cell of an organism. The innate law governs and controls every tissue cell of that unique organism which in turn is expressing its instructive information/F. Being non-discrete, the location of the innate law is everywhere within all the tissues of the body. No exception.

In chiropractic, to satisfy the principle of coordination of action of all the parts of the body (Prin. 32), the innate law uses the innate field as its operating system (OS) to adapt and assemble innate impulses. The innate law uses a Central Processing Unit (CPU), which is the physical brain to centralize innate impulses for coordination of activities. Innate impulses are processed in the physical brain as coded instructions that are distributed through nerve-transmitters to the specific parts of the body. Trophic impulses are transmitted for feedback from the parts of the body, as specific output, to the brain-CPU for reprocessing, as long as it is possible according to universal laws (Prin. 24). Thus the initial input (from the innate law) transmitted from the brain-CPU to the body part receptor and the final output of the body part receptor (also from the innate law) transmitted back to the brain-CPU complete a cycle for coordination of activities.

ART. 34. CYCLES

The Merriam-Webster Dictionary defines *cycles* as:

> **1:** An interval of time during which a sequence of a recurring succession of events or phenomena is completed

> **2a:** A course or series of events or operations that recur regularly and usually lead back to the starting point

> **2b:** One complete performance of a vibration, electric oscillation, current alternation, or other periodic process

> **2c:** A permutation of a set of ordered elements in which each element takes the place of the next and the last becomes first

The term cycle in chiropractic means a course of series of events or operations that recur regularly and usually lead back to the starting point. It is a circuit from cause to effect and effect to cause. It requires adaptation, characterization, instruction, action, and report. It requires input, processing, computing, output, and a feedback loop.

ART. 35. CHIROPRACTIC CYCLES

One of the many infinite cycles of the body that chiropractic addresses is the course of innate information/F from the physical brain to the respective body part, for coordination of activities and feedback reporting that returns to the physical brain, including the consecutive places and operations to satisfy the principle of coordination (Prin. 32).

This particular cycle that chiropractic addresses is a description of the successive steps from cause to effect and back to cause again. It is the hard to vary explanation of what happens between cause and effect and effect and cause regarding coordination of activities of all the parts of the body.

The student will notice that everything in the universe is going through cycles according to their properties and actions. Many cycles go on indefinitely, while others may be limited and go for a set period of time (Prin. 24) due to limitation of E/matter. For example, the lifetime of the body of a living thing is limited, the menstrual cycle is limited, red blood cells live a four month cycle and are replaced, etc... The number of cycles in the body is infinite.

The cycle that chiropractic addresses can be explained over and over and over again, going from general to specific and back again. To break it down, we confine ourselves to a hard to vary explanation based on the principles of chiropractic's basic science. A hard to vary explanation is one that "provides specific details about the principles of its basic science that fit together so tightly that it is impossible to change any detail without affecting its whole." A multitude of cycles are going on at the same time. The number of cycles we employ to describe a process is just what we make of it. Some of them might be introduced within our explanation of chiropractic to show specific examples regarding coordination of activities that we wish to study.

When the explanation of chiropractic is repeated many times, it becomes a streamlined narrative that is worth continuing to disseminate over and over and over again. It becomes a set form so that the same terms are used over and over and over again. It becomes the foundational platform of the chiropractic orientation that is the explanation to the public of WHAT chiropractic is, HOW it is practiced, and WHY it does what it does. When the orientation is refined, it is an outline of the hard to vary explanation of chiropractic based on the principles of chiropractic's basic science. It contains the steps of the cycles as studied in chiropractic philosophy. The briefest one is called, the "simple cycle."

ART. 36. THE SIMPLE CYCLE FOR COORDINATION OF ACTIVITIES

The "simple cycle" is the briefest description from cause to effect and from effect to cause. It names six important processes demonstrating how the non-discrete innate law interfaces with discrete E/matter:

EFFERENT PROCESSES:

    1. Characterization (organizing and encoding information/F into innate impulses)

    2. Transmission (distributing innate impulses)

    3. Expression (acting on innate impulses)

AFFERENT PROCESSES:

    1. Feedback (recoding of impressions into trophic impulses)

    2. Transmission (gathering, sending feedback of trophic impulses)

    3. Interpretation (decoding of trophic impulses)

Notice that transmission occurs twice in this cycle, going from CPU and coming back to CPU. The efferent half denotes the distribution of input of innate impulses from the center. The afferent half denotes a drawing toward the center, a collecting of output actions of feedback from the receptor body part. The innate law adapts information/F by giving it a new character with a new code. This new code characterization becomes innate impulses, which are instructive to the body for coordination of activities of all its parts. It is one way where the union of the non-material with the material aspect of chiropractic occurs, by which the non-discrete innate law maintains discrete E/matter alive for a certain period of time. This link is demonstrated perfectly by the "simple cycle" in Fig. 2 of Art. 38.

ART. 37. THE NORMAL COMPLETE CYCLE FOR COORDINATION OF ACTIVITIES

The "normal complete cycle" applies to the coordination of action of all the parts of the body (Prin. 23). It describes the steps that demonstrate the normal functioning of the innate law (Prin. 27) in order to satisfy the principle of coordination (Prin. 32). This cycle is slightly modified with regard to metabolism and infinitely smaller but no less important, as it happens within every tissue cell. Chiropractic addresses exclusively the correction of vertebral subluxation to restore the transmission of innate impulses. It does not address the radiation of innate rays/waves for metabolism.

In the "normal complete cycle," for coordination of activities only, 31 steps are named, and most of them are processes. The meaning of these steps will be provided later.

Here is the list of the steps:

EFFERENT STEPS:

1. Universal principle of organization
2. Innate law of living things
3. 100%/perfect innate realm
4. Brain cell
5. Characterization/re-organizing
6. Transformation/encoding
7. Innate impulse
8. Propulsion/conductivity
9. Efferent nerve
10. Transmission
11. Tissue cells of body part
12. Reception
13. Physical representation/decoding
14. Expression
15. Function
16. Coordination

AFFERENT STEPS:

17. Tissue cells of body part
18. Vibration
19. Impression/recoding
20. Trophic impulse
21. Afferent nerve
22. Transmission
23. Brain cells
24. Reception
25. 100%/perfect innate realm.
26. Interpretation/decoding
27. Sensation/feedback
28. Integral Innate processes/Interoperability
29. Innate law of living things
30. 100%/perfect instantaneous integral adaptation
31. Universal principle of organization

ART. 38. THE CYCLES GRAPHICALLY REPRESENTED

We will refer to these figures when applicable.

Key for figure 2, 3, 4

BC = Brain Cell	*A= Afferent*	**CPU= Central Processing Unit**		**E =Execute**
TC = Tissue Cell	*E=Efferent*	**R=Receptor**	**D=Decode**	**C=Coordination**

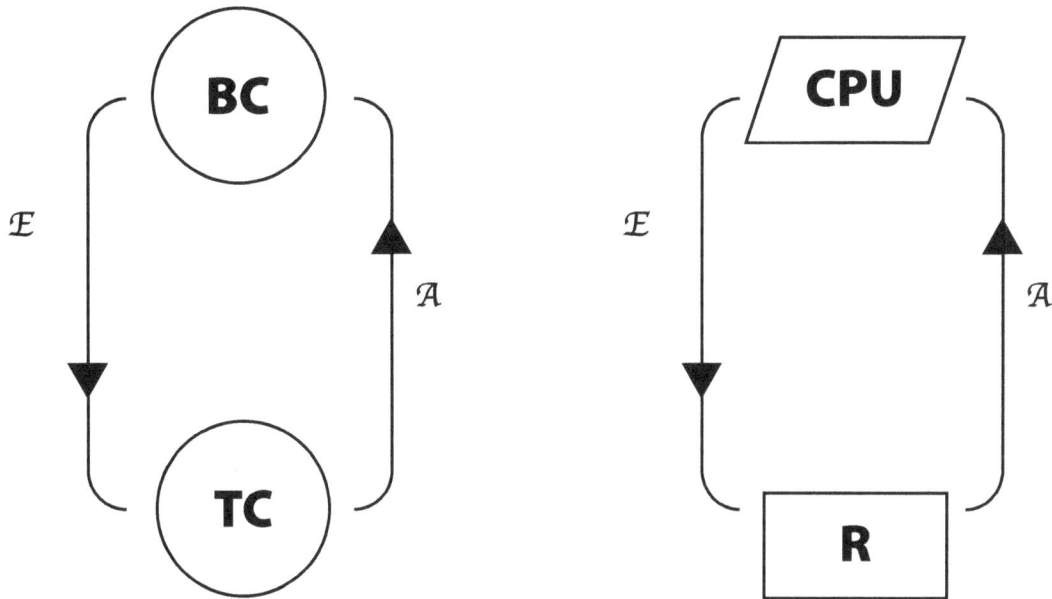

Fig. 2. The "safety pin" cycle is a simple diagram representing the flow of innate impulses from brain cell to tissue cells of the body part for coordination of activities. Regarding the life metabolism of each individual cell, the "safety pin" cycle is occurring through the components of the cell itself. Chiropractic addresses exclusively the interference in transmission for coordination of activities of body parts (Prin. 23, 29, 31).

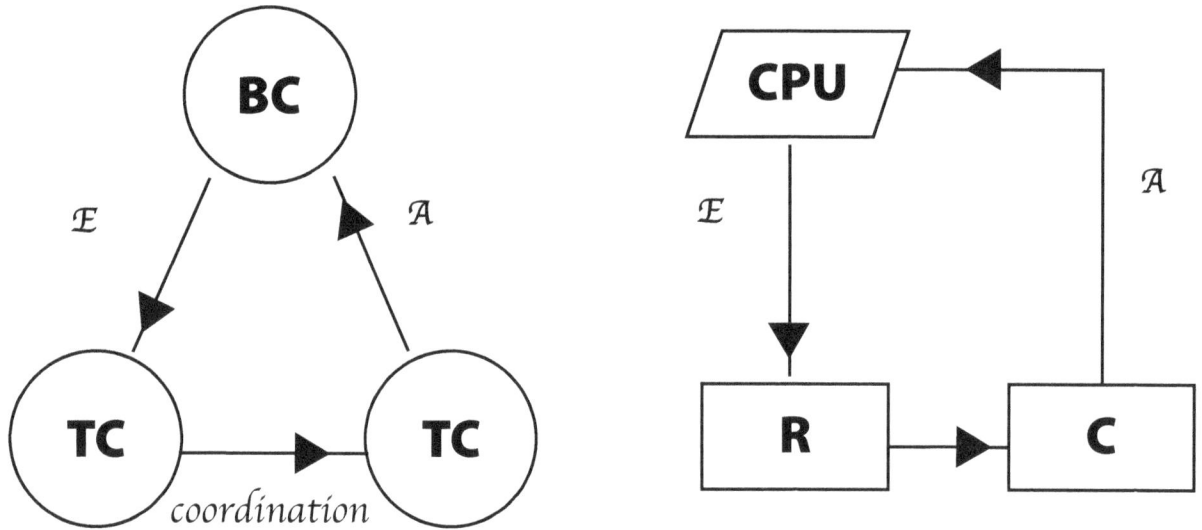

Fig. 3. Simple cycle with the added step of coordination.

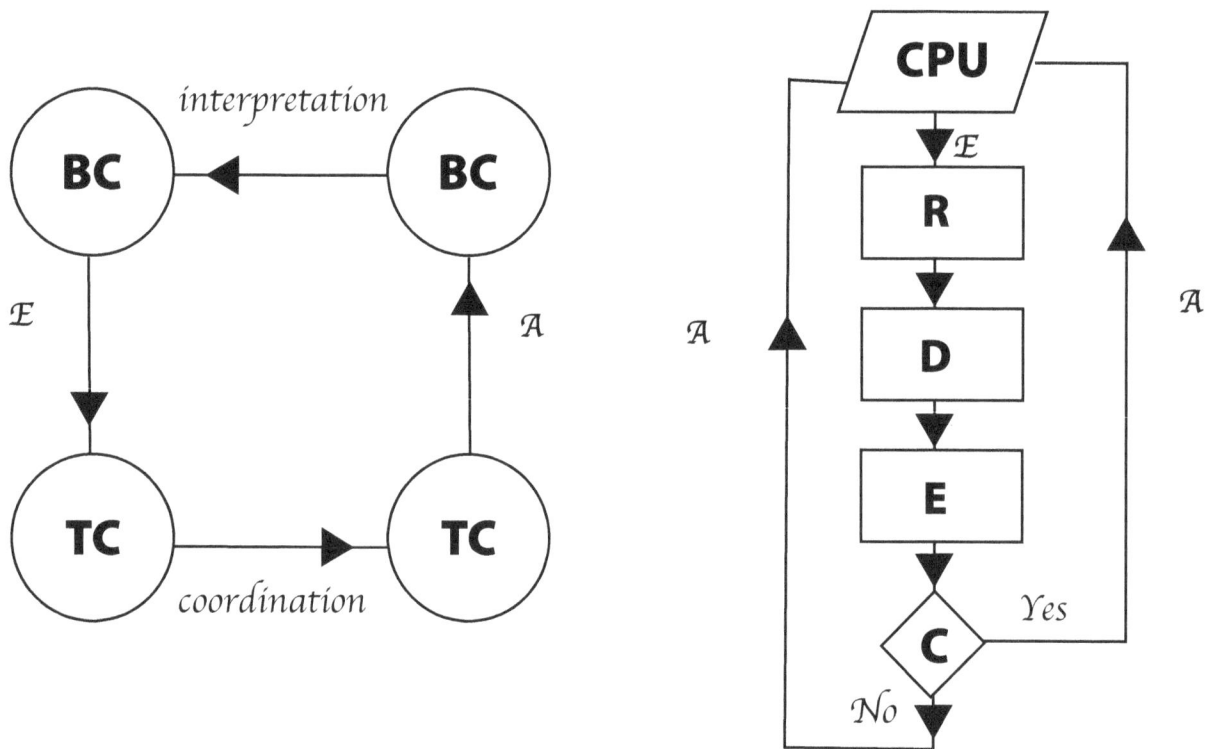

Fig. 4. The simple cycle with an additional step, namely, interpretation/decoding.

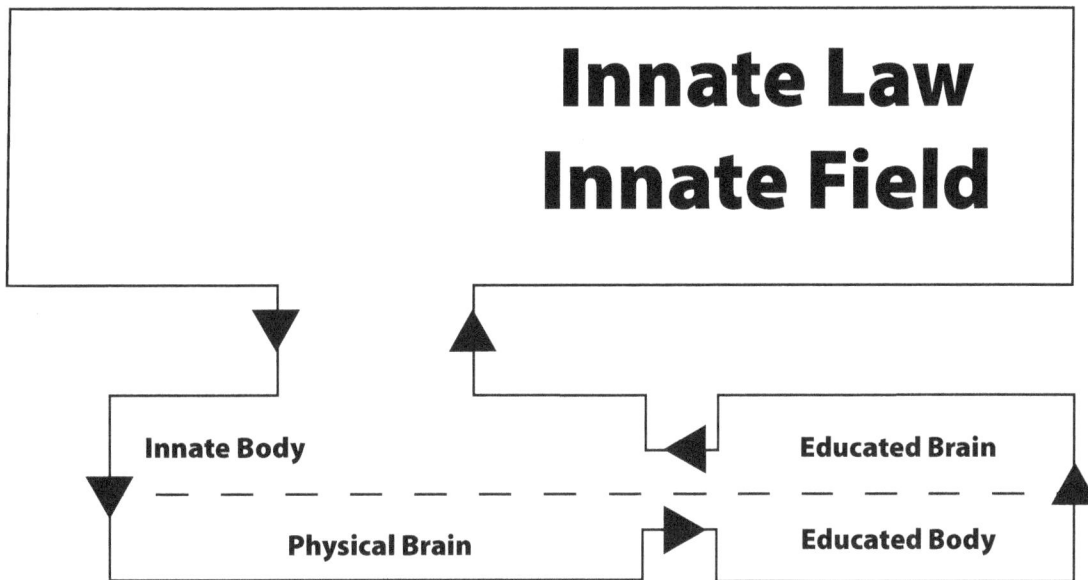

Fig. 5. The "universal diagram of cycles" demonstrating the flow of conducted innate information/F cycles for coordination of activities, which is in units of information/F and E/matter called inforuns (information-force-units from "E=mc² " since energy and matter are interchangeable).

ART. 39. THE NORMAL COMPLETE CYCLE FOR COORDINATION OF ACTIVITIES GRAPHICALLY REPRESENTED

Fig. 6 is a modification of the "safety pin" diagram including the 31 steps of the cycle. It is patterned after its original construct in the Chiropractic Text Book (p.11) called, The Normal Complete Cycle.

When Dr. Ralph W. Stephenson wrote the original chiropractic textbook in 1927, he did not have any knowledge of computer data processing. Therefore, the normal complete cycle for coordination of activities was constructed to demonstrate some arbitrary steps that he organized for teaching purposes using theism and anthropomorphic characteristics (e.g., universal intelligence, mental, creation, physical personification, ideation, innate intelligence). Today, the same steps can be demonstrated through a computer flow chart without theistic or anthropomorphic indicatives.

The Merriam-Webster Dictionary defines *flowchart* as a diagram that shows step-by-step progression through a procedure or system especially using connecting lines and a set of conventional symbols.

A flowchart in chiropractic is a diagrammatic representation of a step by step process of bodily systems. It is a gradual flow of data through information processing systems of body parts. The flow is a set of logic operations under innate control, only if it is possible according to universal laws (Prin. 23, 24). It provides a visual dimension of basic flowchart symbols and their proposed use in a workflow diagram. These are active symbols describing logical steps within the flow of the innate impulse from initial instructions (input) to final actions (output) including feedback for coordination of activities.

1 - Universal Principle of Organization - 31

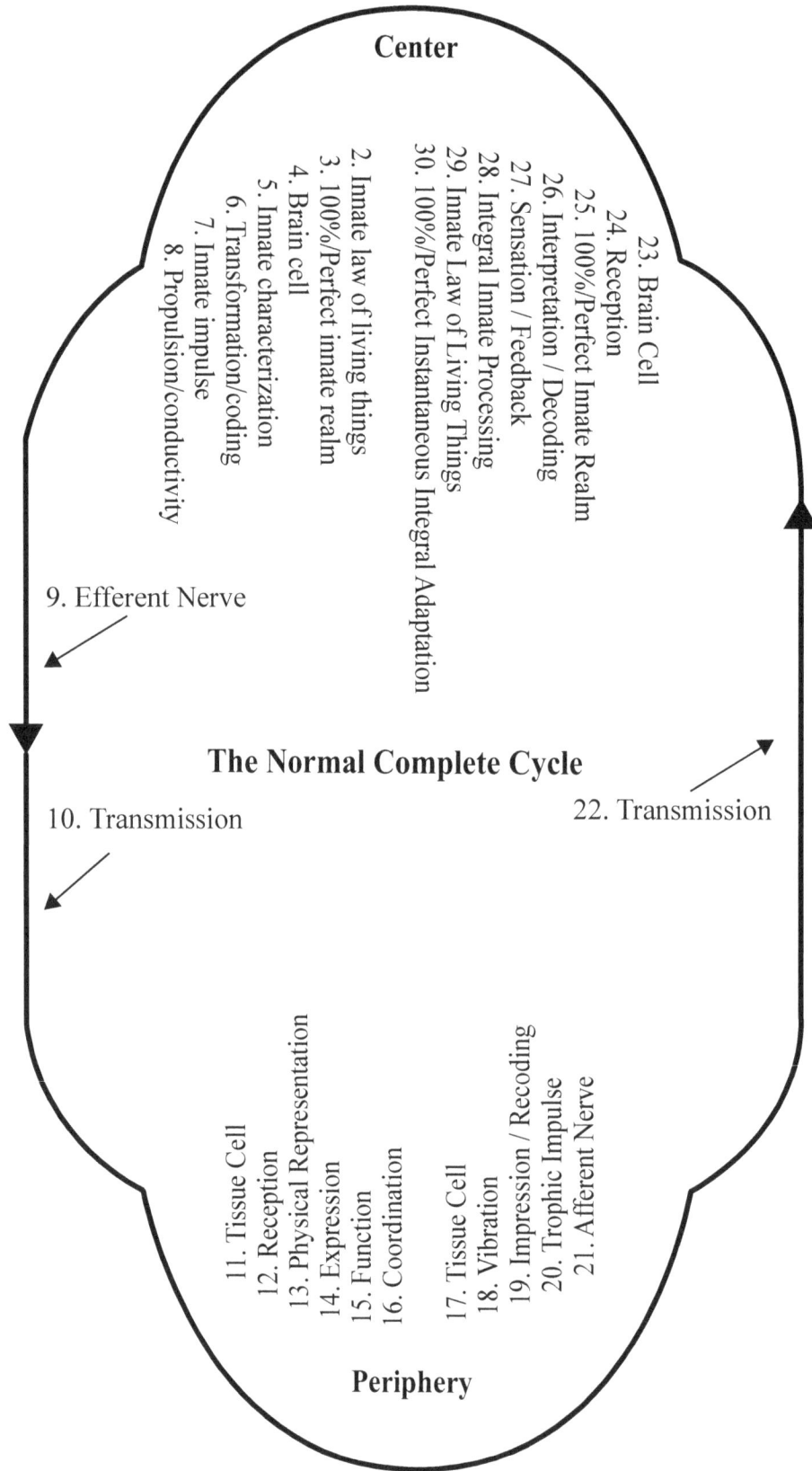

Center

23. Brain Cell
24. Reception
25. 100%/Perfect Innate Realm
26. Interpretation / Decoding
27. Sensation / Feedback
28. Integral Innate Processing
29. Innate Law of Living Things
30. 100%/Perfect Instantaneous Integral Adaptation

2. Innate law of living things
3. 100%/Perfect innate realm
4. Brain cell
5. Innate characterization
6. Transformation/coding
7. Innate impulse
8. Propulsion/conductivity

9. Efferent Nerve

The Normal Complete Cycle

10. Transmission

22. Transmission

11. Tissue Cell
12. Reception
13. Physical Representation
14. Expression
15. Function
16. Coordination
17. Tissue Cell
18. Vibration
19. Impression / Recoding
20. Trophic Impulse
21. Afferent Nerve

Periphery

Fig. 6. The Normal Complete Cycle diagram, demonstrating the 31 steps.

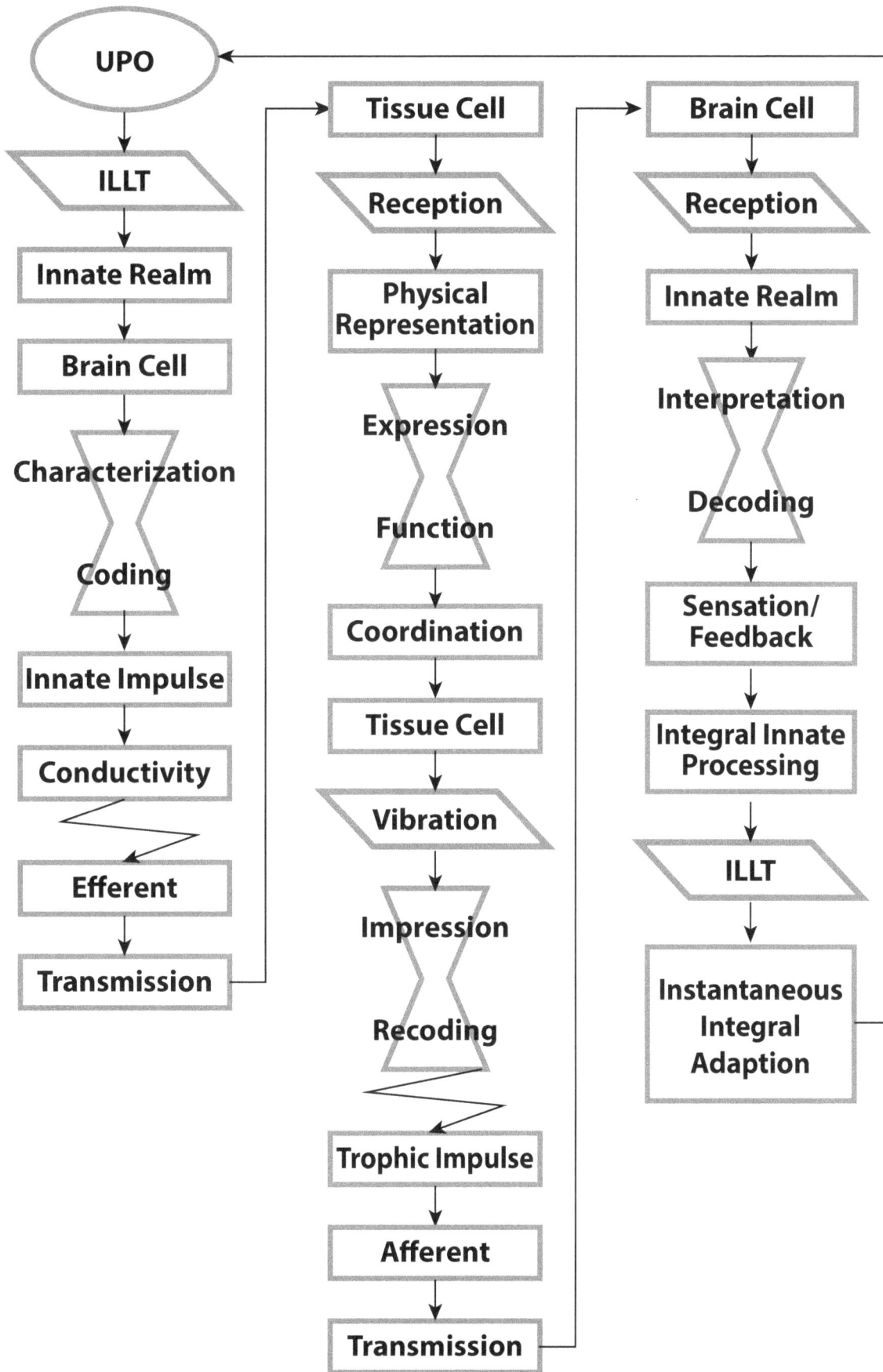

Fig. 7. The 31 steps of the flowchart of the "Normal Complete Cycle."

ART. 40. UNITS

The study chiropractic cycles uses its own unique unit system of information/F and E/matter.

The unit of information/F is the inforun (information/F unit). The unit of E/matter is the tissue cell of the body part inclusive of the physical brain. The smallest unit in function is the tissue cell of the part for coordination of activities. All the steps of the cycle are the names of units of information/F, processes, E/matter, and areas. As the C.G.S. (Centimeter, Gram, Second) is the fundamental unit system in the study of physics, or the I.P.O. (Input, Processing, Output) in the study of computation, so the I.II.TC. (inforun, innate impulse, and tissue cell) is the fundamental unit system in the study of chiropractic. They are terms unique to the chiropractic lexicon.

REVIEW QUESTIONS ARTICLES 32 - 40

1.   What is the Central Processing Unit (CPU) in animal bodies?

2.   Where is the Innate Law of Living Things in the body of living things?

3.   What is a cycle?

4.   What is the one cycle that chiropractic addresses?

5.   How many cycles are there in the universe?

6.   How many cycles are there in the human body?

7.   Why is it necessary to go from the general to the specific in the study of cycles?

8.   Why are the cycles of chiropractic merely names of steps?

9.   Name the steps of the simple cycle?

10. How many steps are there in the normal complete cycle?

11. How many are efferent; how many are afferent?

12. What is the smallest unit of E/matter considered in function?

13. What is an inforun?

14. What is a flowchart in chiropractic?

ART. 41.   THE FUNDAMENTAL CAUSE IN CHIROPRACTIC

The fundamental cause in chiropractic is the capability of the universal principle of organization to organize all of the infinite information/F in the universal field to provide the properties and the actions of E/matter maintaining it in existence (Prin. 1). Chiropractic philosophy asserts that a universal intelligence is the capability of this organizing principle, which is the starting point of chiropractic's basic science, because organization bespeaks intelligence. The student may then ask, "Where does this universal intelligence come from?" This question remains outside the realm of chiropractic philosophy, science, and art. It is a question that belongs to another realm of study. Chiropractic is not theology or spirituality or religion or occultism, etc.

Philosophically in chiropractic we are concerned with a universal intelligence as the fundamental cause of an organizing principle that is necessary to maintain the universe in existence. The universal principle of organization is the initial condition of chiropractic's basic science. This universal principle of organization is a principle that continually organizes information/F, providing properties and actions to all E/matter to be continually maintained in existence. The universal principle of organization is inexhaustible and limitless in its never-ending organization of already existing information/F that provides properties and actions to already existing E/matter. Therefore, the innate law of living things has an unlimited abundance of information/F to adapt to maintain the body of a living thing alive for a lifetime. However, even though the innate law is 100%/perfect, it will always adapt information/F and E/matter for the body only if it is possible according to universal laws (Prin. 24). The innate law is limited by the limitation of E/matter and time.

ART. 42.   THE SALIENT CAUSE OF THE PRACTICE OF CHIROPRACTIC

The salient cause is the immediate adapting information/F for the collection of biological cells to be constructed and maintained alive moment to moment according to universal laws. Chiropractic philosophy identifies this as a salient cause, due to its necessity for the organization and implementation of the rules that govern the body of a living thing. We refer to this "salient" cause as the innate law of living things (Prin. 20). Philosophically speaking, since organization bespeaks intelligence, it has been called the innate intelligence of life. The innate law has been designed by a universal intelligence as an essential continuation of the universal principle of organization that is intrinsic to the increased level of complexity of the body of a living thing. It constitutes biological life. It is the adapted information/F and E/matter expressed by living E/matter (Prin. 13).

We are concerned with it here, philosophically, as an explanation that is hard to vary of a part of the universal diagram. It is called the salient cause of the practice of chiropractic because it is intrinsic and localized only to the body of a living thing, and chiropractic is involved primarily with the living human body. It is a salient law since it is an essential continual extension of the fundamental principle in order to govern the more complex levels of living E/matter. There is no demarcation between the innate law of living things and the universal principle of organization. There is no need, for anything non-discrete is everywhere.

ART. 43. INNATE FIELD

The innate field is that non-discrete aspect of the body that is utilized by the innate law, as an operating system, to adapt, assemble, code, and characterize universal information/F into innate information/F. The innate field is operated by the innate law to assemble innate information/F for use in the body, and for coordination of activities (Prin. 23). It is supplied with innate information/F directly from the innate law. It is the operating system of the innate law to govern everything in the body. It is vital and cannot lack ease since it is 100%/perfect and is non-discrete as is the innate law (Prin. 23). Its location is wherever the innate law is in the body, which is everywhere within the body. The innate field is not only confined to the physical brain of the body for it is everywhere in the body of the living thing. It existence is actual, it is vital, and it is a field that is operated by the innate law.

There is no transmission, radiation or oscillation involved in the supply of innate information/F to the innate field by the innate law. There is no necessity, since they both are non-discrete, they are everywhere within the body. For this reason the innate field always has 100%/perfect innate information/F. This being true, it has 100%/perfect function, and is always congruent with the principle of coordination of action (Prin. 32). It is of course subject to trauma since it interfaces with the body where the non-material unites with the material, the non-discrete with the discrete through innate information/F (Prin. 10). The innate field is a means by which the interaction between the innate law and the interoperability of all body functions is achieved in order for them to be governed. The innate field is the system used by the innate law through which it organizes and assembles information/F uniting itself with living E/matter. This operating system must be supplied with sustenance since it interfaces and interacts with E/matter. The innate field is an interface medium that is a field of operations to assemble innate information/F and is located everywhere within all the tissues of the living body. It is the field of computing operations of the innate law to control and govern, which is why it is called the innate field. What happens in the innate field is always under the control of the innate law. The innate field is the operating system of the innate law for computing and processing everything! Whatever happens anywhere in the innate field is simultaneously experienced everywhere in the innate field. It is the field where the adapting, assembling, characterizing, and coding of constructive information/F happens. It is within innate field that the innate control of the innate law governs every process of the living body, no exception. The innate field will operate on if it is possible according to universal laws; it is limited by the limitation of E/matter (Prin. 24).

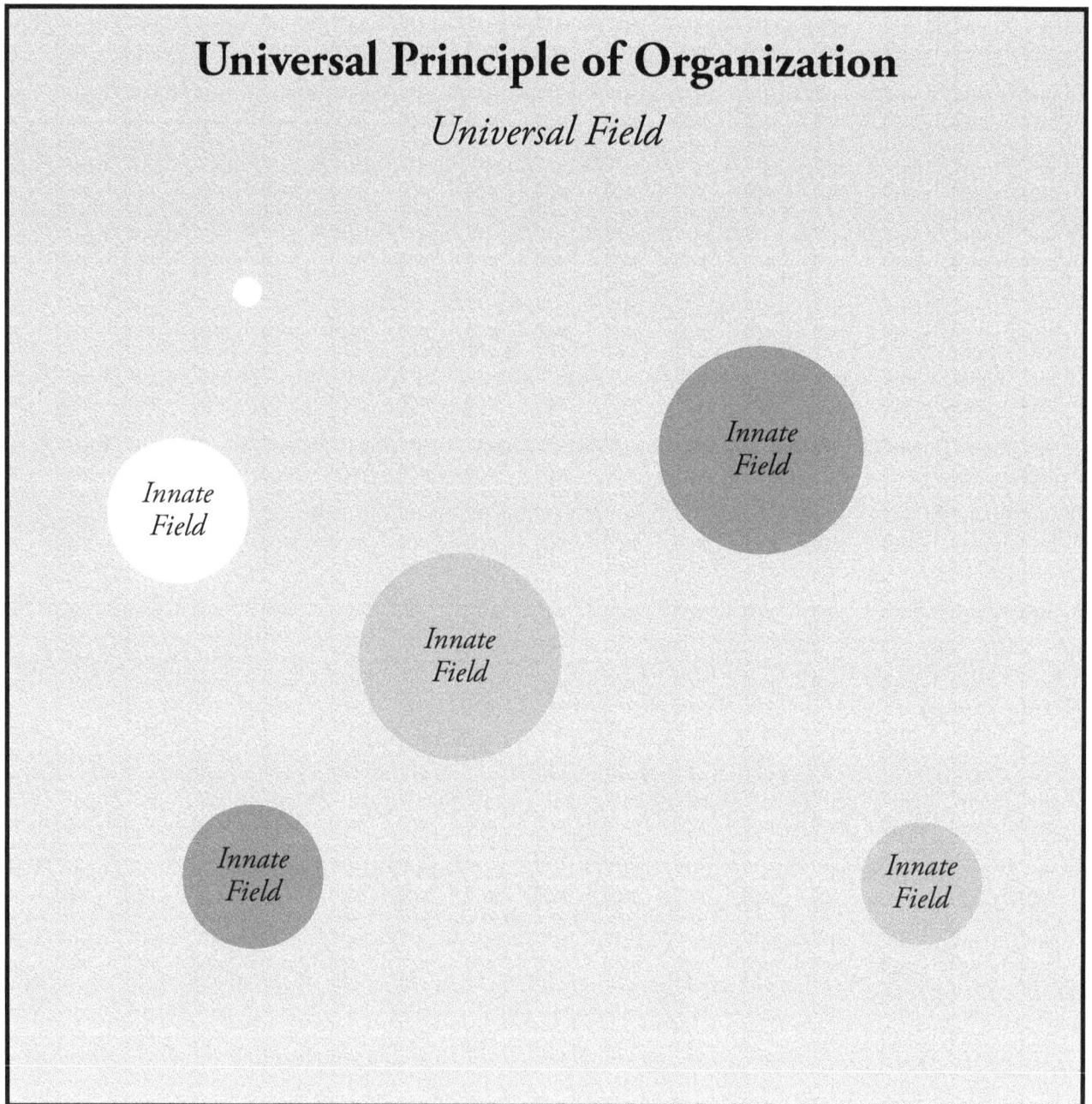

Universal Principle of Organization
Universal Field

Fig. 8. The box indicates ALL existence living, and non-living maintained by the universal principle of organization indicated in regular grey. The innate law of living things is a part of and a part from the universal principle of organization. It is an essential extension of the universal principle of organization designed and programmed by a universal intelligence. It is possible only for living E/matter (and information/F) to be adapted by the innate law, so as to maintain it alive for a lifetime due to the sign of life called adaptability. The degree of adaptation from the innate law is contingent on its level of organization (Prin. 24). Living things are represented as innate fields, governed by the innate law, within existence under the universal principle of organization, part of it, yet distinct. They are varying shades of grey to suit their level of complexity. They are all still grey. Just varying shades of grey to represent various states of living E/matter.

ART. 44. THE EDUCATED BRAIN

It is that part of the physical brain used by the innate law of living things as an organ, for reason, memory, education, conscience, and the voluntary functions, including the will. It is supplied with innate impulses by the innate law. It is subject to lack of ease (DIS-EASE), due to vertebral subluxations directly or indirectly, thus it can have in-coordination of action. It is not vital. It is located within the cerebral cortex of the physical brain. It is the chief organ of adaptation to environmental conditions.

The educated brain is an organ used by the innate law for several specific purposes just as the liver and stomach are used for certain purposes. It is constructed of living E/matter and therefore it has limitations (Prin. 24). Due to this limitation of E/matter, any of its functions can breakdown including thoughts, intuition, instinct, intellectual processing of computation, reasoning, memory storage and retrieval, environmental perceptions and assessments, and "tinctured" innate impulses into educated impulses for conscious voluntary actions that pertain to the will. While breakdown may be due to a multitude of causes, chiropractic addresses only one cause: vertebral subluxation. Vertebral subluxation interferes with the transmission of innate impulses for coordination of activities of body parts (Prin. 23, 31a). It is through the location, analysis, and facilitation of the correction of vertebral subluxations, in accordance with the principles of chiropractic's basic science (Prin. 29, 30, 31), that the chiropractic objective is applied in practice. The practice of the chiropractic objective is nothing more than that, nothing less than that and nothing else than that.

With regards to "tincturing" of innate impulses for voluntary actions, it is a capability of the educated brain of the individual, to imbue a specific character of his/her resolve to an innate impulse that transforms it into an educated impulse to perform a certain voluntary act. For example, the type of muscle responsible for moving your arm to reach for a glass of water is called a voluntary muscle. It is attached to the bones of your shoulder, arm, wrist, hand, and fingers. It moves these bones under your educated control as it receives educated impulses from your educated brain that are conducted through your nerve system. When your educated control stops tincturing innate impulses, the educated impulses are no longer transmitted and the muscles relax and are no longer performing voluntary actions. This voluntary action can only occur because the original innate impulse is an adapted, characterized, and coded universal information/F by the innate law. However, the educated brain then imbues it with a specific new character and transforms it into an educated impulse for voluntary actions. Voluntary actions are accomplished because you use your educated brain to do them.

Therefore, the educated brain possesses a capability to function consisting of a learned versatility that can "tincture" innate impulses that will carry out voluntary actions; it is called educated intelligence (see lexicon). It will be studied in depth in Volume Four.

Note: The student is reminded that the universal principle of organization is the initial fundamental chiropractic principle that is organizing information/F providing properties and actions to all E/matter to be maintained in existence; then for living E/matter, some information/F is adapted by the innate law into innate impulses for coordination of activities of all the parts of the living body; some information/F is adapted into innate rays or innate waves for metabolism for all the cells of the body. In any event, some innate impulses are tinctured by the individual's resolve, utilizing his/her educated intelligence of the educated brain for voluntary actions.

ART. 45. INNATE BODY

The innate body consists of all the tissue cells of the living body. All the cells of the living body are supplied with innate information/F for metabolism and involuntary functions. The innate body is supplied with innate impulses, coded and assembled within the innate field, from the innate law, centralized in the brain (CPU) and distributed through nerves (transmitters) for coordination of activities of body parts. The innate body is also supplied with innate rays/waves, coded and assembled within the innate field, from the innate law, radiated or oscillated from within all the cells of the living body for their respective and specific metabolism.

All the cells of the living body make up the innate body (See Fig. 5). The distinction is according to function, not according to anatomy. All tissues must have innate control for metabolism and even those tissues that are used for voluntary functions. The tissue cells of the systems that have voluntary functions also have involuntary functions at the same time due to their metabolic activities. All cells are under the complete governance of the innate law to be maintained alive through their respective and specific metabolism.

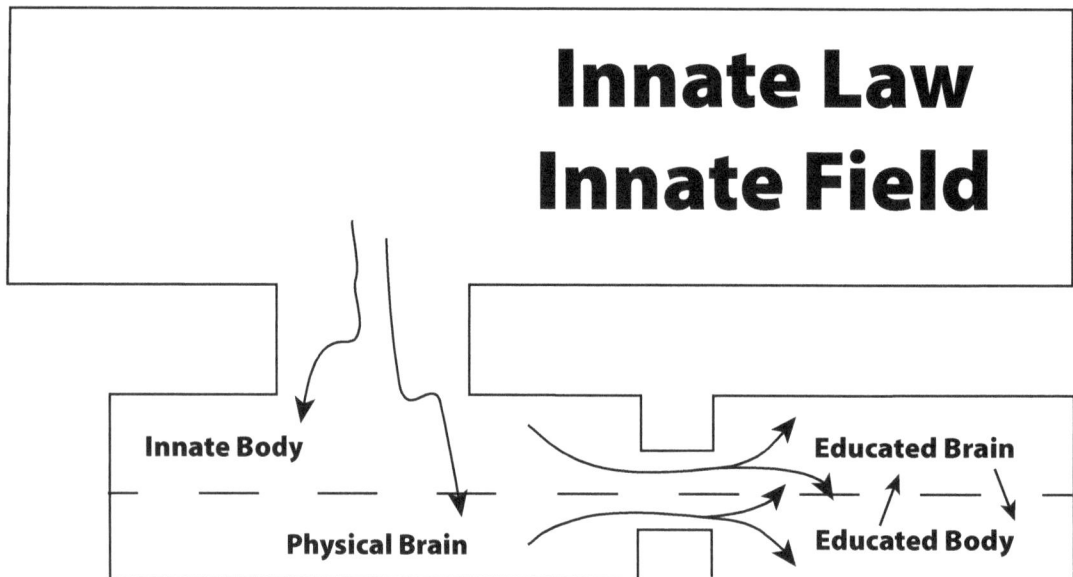

Fig. 9. The "Universal Diagram of Cycles" demonstrates the flow of coded innate information/F that is innate rays radiated and/or oscillated for metabolism, as well as the conducted innate impulses for coordination of activities and the tinctured educated impulses for voluntary actions. Only the conducted innate impulses for coordination of activities will be studied throughout the text since the practice of chiropractic addresses only interference to the transmission conducted innate impulses for coordination of activities (Prin. 29, 30, 31, 32).

ART. 46. EDUCATED BODY

Educated body consists of all the tissue cells supplied with innate impulses from the innate field via the educated brain that have been tinctured into educated impulses for voluntary functions. These same cells are innate body so far as metabolism and the involuntary functions are concerned (See Fig. 5). The distinction is according to function, not according to anatomy. The educated body refers to systems, which can be operated at will (muscles, educated brain and so on), voluntary or conscious movements. Educatedly, the resolve of the individual has no control over the involuntary movements of any tissue cell. Although we may be conscious of some of the involuntary movements that occur in some of the tissue cells, we are unconscious of the metabolism that is happening within these tissues.

ART. 47. INFINITE

According to the Merriam-Webster Dictionary, *infinite* is "extending indefinitely: endless, having no limit. innexaustible. Subject to no limitation."

Universal means everywhere in the universe. If anything is universal it is to be found everywhere; it is in every place and location. The prevailing understanding is that the term universal is an absolute. The universe extends everywhere; it is infinite. It has no limits of space/time, or anything at all. It has no boundaries. This is true of both the material and the non-material universe. The material universe is comprised of E/matter. The non-material universe is comprised of abstractions including a universal intelligence that has designed an organizing principle, which governs every particle of E/matter of the universe. This universal organizing principle manifests many subsequent universal laws and abstractions through the continual organization of information/F that provides the properties and actions of E/matter, thus maintaining it in existence (Prin. 1, 8, 10, 13, 14, 15). The 100%/perfect universe is infinite. Infinite is a descriptive term applied to the universal principle of organization (Prin. 1) and a universal intelligence as its philosophical fundamental cause.

ART. 48. FINITE

According to the Merriam-Webster Dictionary, *finite* is "having definite or definable limits; having a limited nature or existence."

Finite is a term applied to living E/matter because it is maintained alive only for a certain genetic limit of time by the innate law. Therefore, living E/matter is finite according to its lifetime limitations. The nature of the innate law on the other hand, being an essential extension of the non-discrete universal principle of organization, is infinite and adapts living E/matter only if it is possible according to universal laws (Prin. 24). However, universal E/matter is infinite as mentioned in Art. 47, since it is continually maintained in existence by the universal principle of organization. All living E/matter is made of universal E/matter that is adapted by the innate law within the limits of its adaptability. Living E/matter is finite as regards to its being alive for a lifetime. However, it is also infinite regarding its existence since all E/matter is continually maintained in existence by the universal principle of organization. The universal principle of organization and the innate law of living things (which is an essential continuation of the universal principle of organization) are infinite since they both are non-discrete, meaning non-material. It is crucial to differentiate that living things have limits to their lifetime (genetics, hereditary, circumstantial, environmental, etc.) Principle 24 states that the innate law, which is non-discrete and is unlimited, will adapt information/F and E/matter only if it is possible according to universal laws. It is extremely important for us to follow the principles of   chiropractic's basic science, otherwise we risk straying off course from the practice of the chiropractic objective.

ART. 49. THE FIRST STEP OF THE NORMAL COMPLETE CYCLE FOR COORDINATION OF ACTIVITIES: THE UNIVERSAL PRINCIPLE OF ORGANIZATION

Note that the normal complete cycle that is studied in chiropractic concerns only the coordination of activities of the parts of the body. Another cycle (among an infinitude of cycles) is operating as regards to metabolism of the cells of the body (demonstrating interoperability of cell membrane, mitochondria, cilia, lysosomes, centrioles, microtubules, golgi, nucleus, chromatin, ribosomes, cytoplasm, etc.) The practice of chiropractic is not concerned with the cycle of cellular metabolism, even though it can be interfered with by a multitude of causes. The practice of chiropractic is ONLY concerned with restoring transmission of innate impulses for coordination of activities through the correction of vertebral subluxations (Prin. 29, 30, 32).

The universal principle of organization is the infinite organizing principle that maintains everything in existence. This principle is universal and as such, belongs to the universe. Chiropractic appropriates itself of this universal principle of organization, as its initial fundamental principle of its basic science, which is intrinsic to all space/time and E/matter, and which organizes all things, both material and non-material.

The universal principle of organization is inherent to all space/time and E/matter. It is the cause of universal organization. It is 100%/perfect. Organization bespeaks intelligence! Therefore, from a teleological observation, chiropractic philosophy asserts that the universal principle of organization has been designed by 100%/perfect universal intelligence. It cannot err; it is unlimited for it is non-discrete and 100%/perfect. The universal principle organization is the initial condition of chiropractic's basic science. It is not a universal intelligence that is the starting point of the principles of chiropractic basic science. It is the universal principle of organization that is the fundamental principle of chiropractic's basic science; its function is to organize universal information/F continually supplying properties and actions to all E/matter, thus maintaining it in existence (Prin. 1). The universal principle of organization spreads out into an essential continual extension, called the innate law of living things (Prin. 20), as the level of complexity of E/matter increases with novel features of organization of living things. The universal principle of organization extends its continual organizing function into an innate law in order to adapt living E/matter; thus implementing the rules that govern living E/matter and further into thinking E/matter, as infinite manifestations, up the ladder of complexities. Chiropractic acknowledges the universal principle of organization as the beginning of the normal complete cycle, for coordination of activities of the parts of the body of living things. The universal principle of organization is also continually maintaining everything in existence. Without the universal principle of organization existence could not be maintained. Therefore, in chiropractic's basic science, the universal principle of organization is the fundamental starting point, the initial condition of the normal complete cycle. It is the arbitrary first step of the normal complete cycle since it is infinite.

Being an infinite principle, the universal principle of organization cannot be defined. All we can do is get a finite explanation that is hard to vary and formulate an a priori statement based on its manifestation from a teleological observation, which proves its existence through its function, which is universal organization. This a priori statement is the initial principle of chiropractic's basic science. It is a fundamental of chiropractic; it is the initial condition of chiropractic's basis science. The universal principle of organization is a fundamental of the major premise of chiropractic (Prin. 1). Since the universal principle of organization maintains all E/matter in existence, it is also the start of every cycle that exists, including the normal complete cycle for coordination of activities.

ART. 50. THE SECOND STEP OF THE NORMAL COMPLETE CYCLE FOR COORDINATION OF ACTIVITIES: THE INNATE LAW OF LIVING THINGS

The innate law of living things is the inborn organizing principle that controls and governs the body of living things. It is an essential continual extension of the universal principle of organization that is redesigned into an innate law, which is constructing innate information/F to be expressed by living E/matter (Prin. 13, 23, 26). Its purpose is to maintain the body of a living thing alive (Prin. 21). The innate law is the inborn organizing principle intrinsic to living E/matter that is effectively adapting it and information/F to govern its optimization. The innate law is a part of the universal principle of organization and is also distinct from it (Prin. 20)(Fig. 8).

While the innate law is the essential continual extension of the universal principle of organization, it signifies 100%/perfect adaptation, control and governance that the universal principle of organization is expressing through localized more complex living E/matter. All E/matter is maintained in existence by the universal principle of organization, and if it were to cease for one moment, E/matter would cease to exist. This is how the universal principle of organization is the fundamental principle of chiropractic's basic science, its initial condition, and is always continually organizing everything in the universe with 100% of what is required to exist and function. Living E/matter is the evidence of complex organization of the many states of E/matter, which requires adaptation by the essential continual extension of the universal principle of organization called the innate law of living things. Living E/matter specifically requires immediate constant adaptation by the innate law in order to be maintained alive and manifest animate organization, in the form motion (Prin. 14, 15) that evidences the signs of life (Prin. 18). The innate law adapts information/F and E/matter for use in the body so that all parts of the body will have coordination of actions for mutual benefit (Prin. 23).

The Merriam-Webster Dictionary defines *organize* as:

> 1: to form into a coherent unity or functioning whole: INTEGRATE

> 2: to cause to develop an organic structure.

This definition throws an interesting light upon the subject, showing that if a number of interdependent parts are to have a coherent relationship cooperating with each other, they must be grounded about an essential continuous governing control that integrates interoperability. In chiropractic, this governing control is the innate law of living things (Prin. 20) and it reveals the beginning of chiropractic philosophy, in practice, with its hard to vary explanation for the practice of chiropractic. It is the second step of the complete normal cycle for coordination of activities; it is also Prin. 20 of chiropractic basic's science. Therefore, we see that the principles of chiropractic's basic science are clearly the link between chiropractic philosophy and the art of chiropractic. Without guiding principles the philosophy is too vague to be applied through the art.

We notice that there are various states and levels of organization of living things. Some are not much more developed than inorganic E/matter. (See the light circle in Fig. 8). Yet, these are governed by the same 100%/perfect innate law, that is exactly adapting their different levels of organization. These living things are animated perfectly by the innate law according to the specific state of their particular E/matter.

Not only are they maintained in existence by the universal principle of organization, they are maintained alive by its essential continual extension, namely, the innate law of living things, according to universal laws (Prin. 24). This innate law is non-discrete which means non-material, just like the universal principle of organization. It is therefore 100%/perfect for any level of complex organization of E/matter (Prin. 22). Both the shrimp and the whale are governed by the same 100%/perfect innate law (Prin. 7, 20, 21, 22). If it is a living thing, it must be governed by the 100%/perfect innate law in order to be maintained alive according to the limitations of E/matter and time (Prin. 24).

The amount of E/matter of a living thing is limited. The innate law is unlimited. The innate law can adapt an infinite amount of information/F, to be drawn from the whole universe, for use in the body of a particular living thing (Prin. 9). The innate law will adapt E/matter only if it is possible according to universal laws (Prin. 24). The different level of organization of E/matter determines the degree of complexity of its expression of information/F (Prin. 13).

When the body of the living thing has reached its limits of adaptability, its E/matter is not destroyed but it is deconstructed, and reverts back to its elemental state. The innate law is no longer adapting the E/matter of that living thing because the innate law will only do so if it is possible according to universal laws. Since the universal law of genetic lifespan for the body of this particular living thing has reached it limits and has reverted back to a non-living state, the innate law is no longer governing its functions. Again, its E/matter is not destroyed but is deconstructed and reverts back to its inorganic state. It may still be called organic E/matter, as it retains the form of organic E/matter and it still has organic functions at the cellular level during the state of decomposition, but it is no longer alive as far as the body of the living thing is concerned. Most bodily tissues, with the exception of bone, decompose quickly. While the innate law is no longer governing the structures of the body of that particular thing, the universal principle of organization is continually maintaining the fundamental atomic elements of that E/matter in existence through the continuous organizing of information/F that supplies its properties and actions (Prin. 1, 14).

This innate law adapts and assembles E/matter for use in the body constructing it into structures that will be maintained alive without breaking a universal law (Prin. 23, 24). This means that its function is according to a universal design that is programmed by a universal intelligence. It is a localized, innate control that adapts and assembles information/F, from an infinite supply, for self-correction of living structures, through continuous constructive reorganization of living E/matter according to universal laws (Prin. 23, 24). Just as we educatedly adapt gravity, electricity, and heat for our use and convenience, the innate law adapts universal information/F and E/matter for use in the body so that all the parts of the body will have coordinated actions for mutual benefit (Prin. 23). After constructing the structure of the body, the innate law continues to adapt material and information/F to maintain it alive, according to universal laws (Prin. 21, 23, 24).

The distinction between the universal principle of organization and the innate law of living things is that the universal principle of organization continually maintains all E/matter in existence while the innate law of living things maintains living E/matter alive, only for a lifetime, if it is possible according to universal laws. The innate law is limited through the limitations of E/matter and time. This distinction is due to the increasing level of complexity of E/matter that requires adaptation in order to be alive for its lifespan within its limitations (Prin. 24).

Of course, the innate law being the essential extension of the universal principle of organization which is infinite, and which is continually maintaining E/matter in existence, Is also infinite. It cannot be divided. It is just that the innate law is the control that provides rules that governs living E/matter. It is E/matter that is limited and the innate law being 100%/perfect and congruent will not violate its own governing rules. For example, the genetic material of the mayfly is coded and processed by the innate law to construct its structure to live less than 24 hours. The innate law will therefore adapt the body of the mayfly until it reaches its limit of longevity. On the other hand, the genetic material of the Greenland shark is coded and processed by the innate law to construct its structure to live over 270 years. The innate law will adapt the material of the shark, as long as it is possible according to universal laws (Prin. 24). In these two cases, the possibility is the genetic structure of the material of the body of the living thing, its potential adaptability, so it can express innate information/F (Prin. 13). The innate law is always 100%/perfect for all organisms. It does not vary. It is absolute. On the other hand, it is living E/matter that varies in adaptability according to it structural form, its genetic material, and its environmental conditions (as we will demonstrate in the next article). Since vertebral subluxations interfere with transmission of innate impulses, they further increase the limitation of E/matter of the living vertebrate body.

REVIEW QUESTIONS ARTICLES 41 - 50

1. What is the expression fundamental cause synonymous with?

2. What is the expression salient cause synonymous with, and explain that law.

3. What is the innate field?

4. What is the main characteristic of the innate field?

5. What is the educated brain?

6. Does the educated brain govern the body?

7. What is the innate body?

8. What is the educated body?

9. In what "body" are the material cells of the educated body?

10. What does the term universal mean?

11. What do the terms finite and infinite mean?

12. Explain the universal principle of organization, the first step of the cycle for coordination of activities.

13. What is the innate law of living things?

14. What does organize mean?

15. What is the distinction between the universal principle of organization and the innate law of living things?

16. What principle is used as the starting point of chiropractic philosophy that is the platform on which the art of chiropractic is constructed according to this cycle?

17. What is the link between the philosophy and the art in chiropractic?

ART. 51. THE INNATE LAW IS INTRINSIC TO ALL LIVING THINGS

Whenever molecules and atoms have been constructed into cell structures by the instructive information/F of the innate law, the cells are called living E/matter. While animated and actively alive, it is this innate law (which is the inborn organizing principle of living E/matter) that controls and governs those living cells.

Living things extend through a wide range of complex organizational states of E/matter. All living things must have, at least one sign of life in order to be alive (Prin. 18). Some living organisms possess so very little animate organization that it is sometimes very difficult to distinguish these living things from inanimate structures. Yet, the mere fact that they are alive requires 100%/perfect control and governance by the intrinsic innate law (See the thin line circle in Fig. 8).

Complex or simple, spanning through all levels, humans, animals, birds, fish, reptiles, insect, plants, or unicellular organisms, all living things are controlled and governed by the intrinsic innate law. The broadest outlook forms of those organisms comprised of organized and adaptive living E/matter requires extended adaptation from the innate law. This is due to more complex motion and adaptability of the living E/matter within its environment. It is not necessarily dependent on quantity of E/matter. Some unicellular living organism can adapt to some challenging environments, while the more complex organisms cannot. For example, a deep-sea jellyfish of about half-inch size can be found at depths of 3,000 ft adapting very well to its extreme environment, while a 500 lbs dolphin can dive at no deeper than 1,000 ft The same can be said for a 300 lbs lion that will adapt to a temperature of 120°F and will not survive at -40°F, while a 300 lbs polar bear will adapt to -40°F and will not survive at 120°F.

According to the principles of chiropractic's basic science, life is studied generally and specifically. More exactly, existence and viability can be looked at as contrasted phases. All E/matter has existence, which is the motion of its elemental particles (Prin. 14, 15). Viability is the capability of E/matter to live. From a global perspective, the development of chiropractic science and philosophy contends with complex systems, extending from multi levels of organizations of E/matter of divided to condensed non-living E/matter, to adaptive living E/matter, on to thinking living E/matter, up the ladder of complexity. Keep in mind that the practice of chiropractic is concerned only with vertebrates, mainly humans and a variety of domestic animals, since it addresses only vertebral subluxations.

ART. 52. THE THIRD STEP OF THE NORMAL COMPLETE CYCLE FOR COORDINATION OF ACTIVITIES: 100%/PERFECT INNATE REALM

It is the plane activity of the innate law. It is a non-material realm. It pertains to the space where the innate law controls and governs the organization of living E/matter through instantaneous integral adaptation. It is a non-discrete field of activity and is strictly abstract. It is the realm of innate activity, which means that it is where the innate law is computing and processing (Prin. 33). The innate law, as a part of the universal principle of organization, is the adapting law of life, which continuously reorganizes information/F and E/matter within the limits of adaptation (Prin. 24). From chiropractic philosophy, we understand that organization bespeaks intelligence. Therefore, a universal intelligence which is 100%/perfect (Prin. 5) designed and programmed the universal principle of organization which is also 100%/perfect and complete. Intrinsic to the design of the universal principle of organization is a program of unlimited computation that continually organizes boundless and infinite information/F within the universe regardless of environmental conditions.

The function of the universal principle of organization is to continually organize information/F that provides properties and actions to all E/matter to maintain it in existence and also through its essential continual extension, the innate law of living things, to maintain exclusively living E/matter alive according to universal laws (Prin. 1, 8, 21, 24). Anything that is maintained in existence is continually organized by the universal principle of organization (Prin. 1), and anything that is maintained alive is instantaneously adapted by the innate law of living things, according to universal laws (Prin. 20, 21, 23, 24). The process of universal organization and innate adaptation is called characterization, which is the construction and computation of specific codes by the universal principle of organization that organizes universal information/F. It is also the reconstruction (modified codes for living E/matter) of specific instructive information/F by the innate law that adapts universal information/F to assemble into innate information/F. All E/matter must have a certain character to be continually maintained in existence. It also must have an added and modified character (modifier) in order to be maintained alive for a lifetime according to universal laws (Prin. 24).

Every abstract fact, every design, every structure, every act of every part of the body, or the body as a whole, is first computed and assembled in the innate field of the living thing by the 100%/perfect innate law (Prin. 22). Remember, the innate field is that non-discrete aspect of the body that is utilized by the innate law, as an operating system. It is where the innate law adapts, assembles, computes, codes, and characterizes universal information/F into innate information/F. It is part of the innate realm. The innate field is operated by the innate law to assemble innate information/F for use in the body and for coordination of activities (Art. 43 and Prin. 23). It is the operating system of the innate law as a 100%/perfect innate "software." The adapted, computed, and coded characterization of the innate information/F begins in the non-material realm, the non-discrete area, which is wherever the innate law operates, which is everywhere in the body. It is then centralized in the physical brain, as innate impulses, to be conducted through nerves for coordination of activities. It is also radiated and oscillated, from within the cell for metabolism as innate rays or innate waves. The student is reminded that the practice of chiropractic concerns itself exclusively with interference in transmission of innate impulses through the location, analysis, and facilitation of vertebral subluxations. The activity of the universal principle of organization is to continually organize information/F to maintain E/matter in existence (Prin. 1). The activity of the innate law is to adapt (reorganize) information/F and E/matter to maintain living E/matter alive, for a lifetime (Prin. 21, 24). The activity of the universal principle of organization and its essential continual extension, the innate law of living things, is called control of organization. It is an important phase of life that is not overlooked by chiropractic. The student is cautioned to remember that control and governance of organization is not a principle but the activity of principle.

ART. 53. INNATE CONTROL

The term innate control is the activity of the innate law in the innate field. It is the introduction of innate instructions, as governance, into E/matter via the innate field. Chiropractic maintains that the innate law is the dynamic process of computation that is a local activity that controls and governs the body a living thing. It is an intrinsic necessity for the body to live. It explains the emergence of complex patterns in a homogeneous medium, the body of a living thing. In general, the emergence of complex patterns and structures is explained by diversity and adaptability in living E/matter. Without the innate law, E/matter is not maintained alive at all. The term innate control is strictly a chiropractic term (See lexicon.) It is consistent with chiropractic philosophy and it signifies the complete absolute governance of the innate law of the body of living things (Prin. 20, 21).

Innate control is the term applied to what the innate law does when it performs its computation work for adaptation. It is the 100%/perfect dynamic processing of data that adapts information/F and E/matter (Prin. 23). Innate control and educated control (for voluntary actions) are chiropractic terms used to indicate the kind of computation being done. When the innate law is not performing its computation and processing, there is no innate control, no life at all. It is an indicator that living E/matter is deconstructed and reverted back to its basic elements of universal E/matter. It is now non-living E/matter which always continues to exist under the governance of the universal principle of organization.

Let us use some analogies:

Compare a music director to the innate law, his stage to the innate field, his orchestra to the body, and music to the dynamic process of innate control. When the director gives instructions to his orchestra as a body of expression, there is the music of the symphony. When the director ceases to instruct there is no music expressed as the symphony.

 Compare a professor teaching from home using her computer. The professor is comparable to the innate law, her computer is comparable to the brain, her instructions are comparable to innate control. When the professor inputs instructions in her computer, as an agent of expression, there is teaching. When the professor ceases to input there are no instructions expressing the lesson as output.

Compare a pilot to the innate law, the airspace to the innate field, his airplane to the body, his gentle inputs commanding the airplane to the innate control. When the pilot inputs commands to the airplane there is flight. When the pilot ceases to input instructions to the airplane it will stop flying. There is no more output.

In all of these examples, it is the activity of the music director, the professor, or the pilot that is the control of the process.

The activity of the innate law in the innate field of the body is the innate control. The product of this activity is innate information/F such as innate impulses, innate rays or innate waves. This is the interface from a purely non-discrete phenomenon. It is the step necessary to unite the non-material and the material. It is a transitional step to the physical impulse carrying a non-physical instruction. The innate information/F is instruction to living E/matter so it can perform its function, whatever it is at the moment. Innate control is the act of assembling information/F in the innate field. Even when the educated brain is selected as the organ of expression for voluntary actions, the innate information/F must first be assembled in the innate field (See Fig. 5 and Prin. 23).

 As a further point of clarification, the term thought has been used extensively in chiropractic due to its past anthropomorphic tone. It is a term that describes the product of thinking. The prevailing understanding of 100 years ago was that "thought" only occurred in the educated brain. However, Dr. B.J. Palmer while developing chiropractic philosophy went a step further. He personified the innate law. He assigned human characteristics to this scientific law. He mentioned often, in many Green Books, that he was having "thought flashes coming through from Innate," that "she" was his guide, "she" was doing the thinking and that he was simply following her biddings. B.J. Palmer chose to explain the wisdom of the body in anthropomorphic terms. It was how B.J. Palmer understood the workings of the law of life. It was based on the knowledge that was available to him in those days. He was also influenced by the context of his times as well as his own personal intuitions. It was how B.J. chose to develop chiropractic. There have been many guesses as to why B.J. personified "Innate." Whatever the reason, despite the inaccuracies of depicting the innate law in this manner, it is my humble opinion that without B.J.

Palmer, chiropractic could not have developed into what it is today, a simple unadulterated humanitarian approach to life.

It was not until 1973, at Sherman College of Chiropractic in Spartanburg, S.C., that some chiropractors began to see that anthropomorphism was, according to the prevailing understanding of the day, simply a way to speak of the wisdom of the body that could not be otherwise explained. It was the personification of an intangible non-discrete, non-material principle. Today, according to the new information and knowledge that is available, the new understanding is, first and foremost, that the innate law is a scientific, inborn organizing principle (Prin. 20). The innate law is intrinsic to the body of all living things in order to maintain it alive through its 100%/perfect control, according to universal laws (Prin. 21, 23, 24). It is designed and programmed by a universal intelligence. We must always keep in mind that, through teleological observations, 100%/perfect organization bespeaks 100%/perfect intelligence (Prin. 5, 22).

As we refine the chiropractic concepts, we acknowledge that thoughts are part of our nature as human beings. However, thoughts do not only occur in the educated brain. "Thoughts occur not only in the brain but in a tangled communication among brain, body and environment."[13]

For example, say one has the thought "I need water, I'm thirsty." That's because parts of their body were simultaneously instructed, by some computations of the innate law, to produce certain chemicals in their body, perhaps due to environmental factors (such as it is hot outside). Their brain cells made a chemical called angiotensin-2 that, in turn influenced their behavior in such a way that they started looking for a bottle of water. At the same time, their hypothalamus also made a chemical called angiotensin-2, which caused the secretion of a hormone called ADH, which made their body hold on to water to keep within balance. Their heart cells also generated angiotensin-2 so they held on to water. Their kidney cells made angiotensin-2 so they didn't lose water in the urine, and their skin cells produced angiotensin-2 because they need water. The thought "I'm thirsty" did not emerge first in the brain, it is simultaneously produced everywhere in the whole body. Each cell gets the thought at the same time, even though we may think we get it first in the brain. The new notion nowadays is that the act of thinking thoughts has escaped not only the confine of the physical brain, but that "thought" is not even confined to our bodies; it is everywhere in the environment, in all of space/time, all at the same time. Not only do we have a thinking body controlled and governed by the innate law, this thinking body is part of a thinking universe maintained in existence and controlled by a universal principle of organization, which has been designed by a 100%/perfect universal intelligence. We think big. We think out loud. We think outside the box. We think on our feet. But what we don't do is think entirely and only inside our heads. Thoughts are not confined to our brains only. They course through a network that expands to our whole body. The prevalent idea in scientific research today points to something far deeper and more radical. It's not just that our bodies influence thoughts, it's that "thought" itself is a system that simultaneously takes place in the brain, the body and the environment around us. It was the French philosopher Rene Descartes who once said, "cogito ergo sum." I think, therefore I am. With today's new knowledge of embodied cognition, it may very well be a slightly different philosophy: "I am, therefore I think."

Suffice it to say that "thinking" in chiropractic is a term that is not ascribed to the innate law, but a term that is ascribed to the educated intelligence, which is the capability of the educated brain to function. It is not used in reference to the innate law nor should it be used that way. It is a learned process. The process of thinking may still appear to us to be purely non-material, however the evidence points to something quite material. From a very broad perspective, the development of educated intelligence is continually moving toward greater understanding of complex systems of organized and adaptive

---

13. Wilson, A.D., Golonka S. "Embodied cognition is not what you Think it is." Front Psychol. 2013; 4:58 Published 2013 Feb 12.

E/matter, which is material, on to thinking E/matter, which is also material, up the ladder of complexity. When it concerns the function of the innate law, however, adaptation is not a learned process. It is a specific moment-to-moment 100%/perfect adaptive computation. The term that describes its product is innate information/F, which is instructive to the material of the body. It becomes an expressed output from E/matter (Prin. 13) computed from an adapted input (Prin. 23) according to universal laws (Prin. 24). The innate law is basically an unlimited 100%/perfect and normal software, designed, and programmed by a universal intelligence, capable of computing infinite possibilities and potentialities according to universal laws.

ART. 55. EDUCATED CONTROL

Educated control is the activity of the innate law in the educated brain as an organ. The product of this activity is voluntary actions, such as reasoning, will, memory, movements, etc. It is always the innate law that adapts information/F and E/matter for use in the body, including the voluntary organs and systems (Prin. 23). Some of the innate information/F will be tinctured by the educated intelligence through the educated brain for voluntary actions (See Fig. 9). For example, it is important to note that we should not know how to operate the special sense organs even though we can will them to act. The operations of the sense organs are an innate control. Their functional use is an educated control. Educated information/F is mostly for adaptation to the environment.

ART. 56. THE FOURTH STEP OF THE NORMAL COMPLETE CYCLE FOR COORDINATION OF ACTIVITIES: BRAIN CELL

The brain (CPU) is an organ used by the innate law to centralize innate information/F that has been assembled in the innate field to be conducted through the nerves for coordination of activities. The innate law is intrinsic to all tissue cells of the body. The innate information/F that will be conducted through nerves for coordination of activities emanate from the physical brain, which is the central processing unit for distribution. It is where innate impulses are continuously computed for coordination of actions of all the parts of the body according to universal laws (Prin. 23, 24). As the brain is an organ, so is the brain cell a smaller unit. The brain cells form the structure of the CPU where the innate law centralizes the innate impulses to be conducted through the nerves for coordination of activities. Metabolically, it is a tissue cell requiring innate information/F, blood, and serum.

A brain cell is a cell of nerve tissue – one of the four primary tissues. It has many properties of other tissue cells, having a body and a nucleus. It is called a neuron or a glia. However, a neuron has a unique architecture compared to other tissue cells. According to NIH, "a neuron has three basic parts: a cell body and two extensions called an axon and a dendrite. Within the body of the cell is a nucleus, where the cell's activities take place and it contains the cell's genetic material. The axon looks like a long tail and transmits messages from the cell. Dendrites look like the branches of a tree and receive messages from the cell. The glial cells support the neurons in their work; they are called astrocytes and oligodendrocytes"[14]

Axons bundle up forming the spinal cord, extending from the brain down through the spinal canal. They branch and subdivide to all parts of the body for coordination of actions (Prin. 23, 28). The brain and spinal cord make up the central nerve system. The nerves are called the peripheral nerve system.

---

14. "Brain Basics: The Life and Death of a Neuron." https://www.ninds.nih.gov/health-information/public-education/brain-basics/brain-basics-life-and-death-neuron#:~:text=A neuron has three basic,sends messages from the cell June 2023

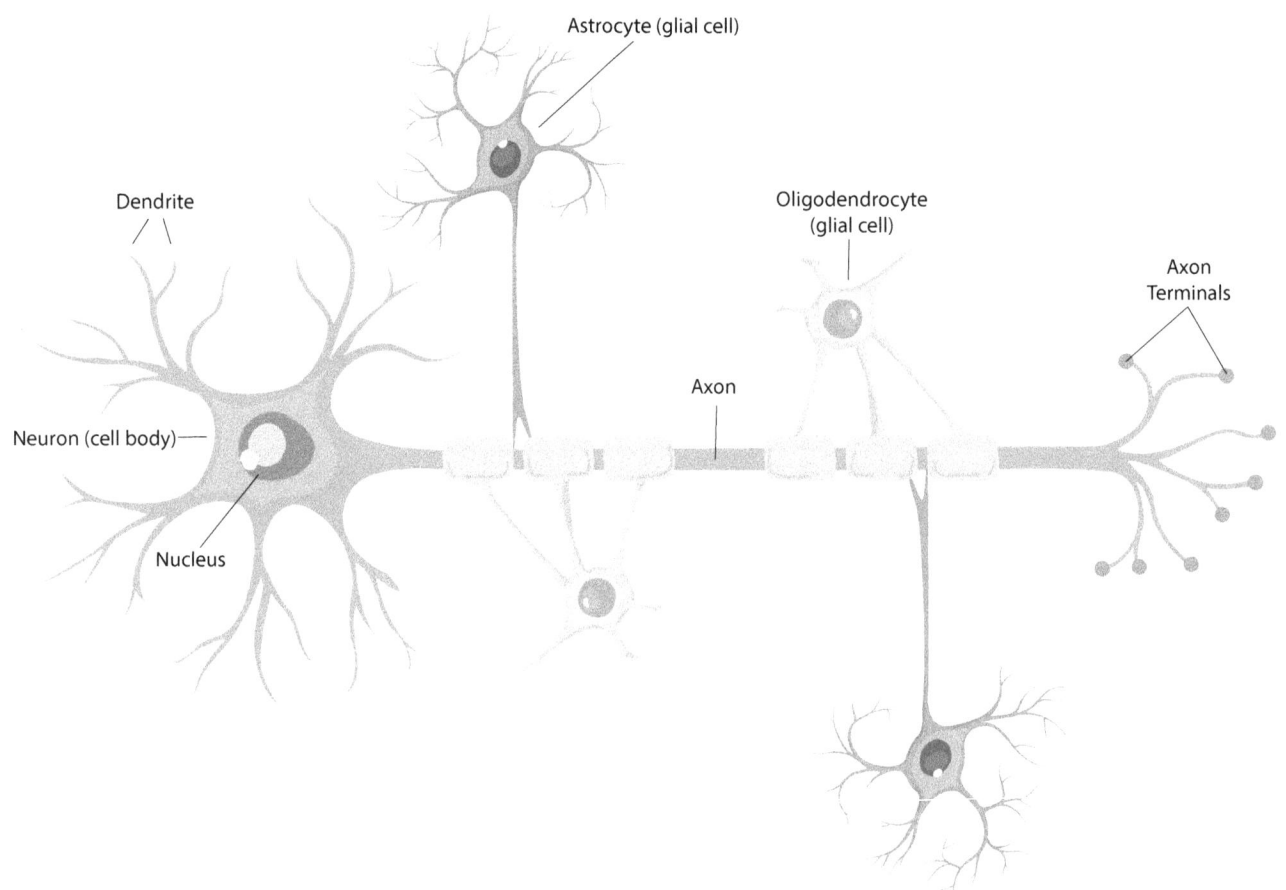

Fig. 10. Diagram demonstrating the parts of the neuron.

ART. 57. THE FIFTH STEP OF THE NORMAL COMPLETE CYCLE FOR COORDINATION OF ACTIVITIES: INNATE CHARACTERIZATION

Innate characterization/coding is the process of adapting universal information/F in the innate field, so that it can be used for the maintenance and functioning of tissue cells including coordination of activities of all body parts (Prin. 8, 23, 28). It is the reorganizing and assembling of information/F in the innate field, by the innate law, that will emerge from the physical brain to be centralized and conducted for coordination of activities; or that will emerge from all other tissue cells and to be radiated and/or oscillated for metabolism of the tissue cells (that includes also the brain cells.) This emergence of adapted innate information/F within tissue cells is the interface where transformation will occur. According to the Merriam-Webster dictionary, *characterization* is derived from "caracter, from Latin character mark, distinctive quality." Again, according to Merriam-Webster, *code* is "a system of signals or symbols for communication."

Innate characterization/coding in the innate field refers to the adapting, reorganizing, and assembling of something, already characterized by the universal principle of organization. It is a characterization/coding done in a certain way. It is really a re-characterization/coding of universal information/F into innate information/F in the innate field. It is the innate law that is investing information/F with a new character/code suitable to living E/matter to be maintained alive, (Prin. 21, 23) for its lifetime according to universal laws (Prin. 24). Universal information/F already exists and is continually organized by the universal principle of organization to maintain the existence of E/matter (Prin. 1). Of course, there is adapting, reorganizing, and assembling of innate information/F that is constructing a multitude of complex organizational states of E/matter into living structures. Any builder, for example, assembles building materials into structures and assembles different subcontractors to organize and accomplish the work. This is how building materials become characterized according to the specific forms of the structure that is being constructed. Planks of wood and glass panes are sculpted in certain shapes, spools of wires are cut and twisted in certain ways, piles of pipe are fitted in specific length, etc. All materials are characterized and assembled according to specific architectural designs. The innate law cannot deconstruct E/matter to its elemental particles; neither can it function contrary to universal laws (Prin. 24, 25, 26, 27). However, the 100%/perfect innate law can adapt, reorganize, employ, diminish, augment, transform, and assemble the information/F and E/matter that is necessary to accomplish the constructive ends that maintains the body alive, according to universal laws (Prin. 21, 23, 24).

The innate law is also a 100%/perfect software using the innate field as its operating system to adapt and assemble innate information/F. It is in this sense that the term characterization/coding is used in the normal complete cycle for coordination of activities. Universally, characterization/coding is the continuous computation of information/F by the universal principle of organization, intrinsic to all E/matter that has been designed and programmed by a universal intelligence. The universal principle of organization continually maintains all of E/matter (living and non-living) in existence (Prin. 1). For example, when Fig. 8 was constructed, the size of the circles, the shade of grey, the letters, the lines, were all existing as components of the computer software. Those abstract signs were re-characterized into meaningful visuals adapting them to figuratively represent the content of the text as an imagined image.

Remember that the innate characterization/coding is accomplished according to the organizational complexities of the living E/matter that is being adapted moment to moment to its internal and external environment. As we arbitrarily jump into this cycle, we must always realize that, it only concerns coordination of activities related to the practice of chiropractic. For example, if we study the coming of the season of spring, we learn that it comes as a result of waters from rivers and streams that are producing moisture for vegetation growth. We understand, however, that water came from an earlier step in the cycle, the melting of snow from the previous winter. Each successive step is dependent upon the previous one. Innate characterization/coding is dependent upon the previous step, which is the 100%/perfect innate realm where universal information/F is adapted by the innate law. In order to have coordination of activities, the innate law (100%/perfect software) that is intrinsic to living E/matter, must first adapt, assemble, and characterize/code information/F to be conducted as innate impulses and transmitted from the brain through the nerves, according to universal laws (Prin. 23, 24, 28, 32).

ART. 58. THE SIXTH STEP OF THE NORMAL COMPLETE CYCLE FOR COORDINATION OF ACTIVITIES: TRANSFORMATION/ENCODING

Transformation is the encoding step where innate information/F is modified, converted and reconstructed into a specific unit. It is converted and reconstructed information/F from the innate realm to the material realm. It is the encoding of inforuns (See lexicon) by the 100%/perfect software program, which is the innate law, that are organized and continually maintained in existence by the universal principle of organization, for use in the tissue cell. This step includes the modification of information/F into an innate impulse that instructs living E/matter to act for coordination of activities (Prin. 23). It is encoding innate information/F with specific instructions, through 100%/perfect innate processing, moment by moment, so that it can be expressed in physical forms (Prin. 13).

Transformation/encoding is the most difficult process of the cycle to understand. The innate law is always acting according to what's going on in the body of the living thing and its environment moment by moment. It will adapt information/F and E/matter only if it is possible according to universal laws (Prin. 24). When the innate law assembles universal information/F in the innate field, they are already part of a universal field of unlimited possibilities and potentialities. This is literally a field, in so far as if the field is stimulated anywhere, it is experienced in the whole field everywhere. This universal field is the operating system of the universe controlled by the universal principle of organization. Universal information/F is continuously computed and organized by the universal principle of organization (Prin. 8). The universal principle of organization has been designed by a universal intelligence. In this non-specific state universal information/F is called inforuns. It is, as yet, the most specific instructions from the universal principle of organization to control infinite possibilities and potentialities of the universe, and they are absolutely abstract and non-discrete (See lexicon.) In this universal field, these instructions are part of all of space/time. The already 100%/perfect universe (Prin. 5) is maintained in existence by the universal principle of organization that is intrinsic to all E/matter continually providing its properties and actions (Prin. 1) through the organization of information/F (Prin. 8). Information/F unites the universal principle with E/matter (Prin. 10) and reveals the interface between the organizing principle and E/matter. It is the link between the non-material and the material. Transformation/encoding is the process of modifying these inforuns to become innate information/F that are instructions for maintaining living E/matter alive according to universal laws. It really is the interface that is the link between the non-material and the material. Anyone using a cell phone sees that there is instructive information built into its software, which is the interface allowing communication between users. This software is abstract information in the form of a program language comprised of signs and symbols. There is no tangible connection between the users that are miles apart, yet they are united through electromagnetic waves that are intangible, but are by no means abstract, in the sense that possibilities and potentialities are theoretical.

In the same way, the human body is a device that human beings use to relate and communicate with each other and the environment. You are not your body. If you lose a finger or an eye, you are still the same you. It is your body device that's missing something, not you. The internal software running your body device is 100%/perfect and never ever needs updating. It always computes with perfect accuracy moment by moment all potentialities and possibilities within universal laws (Prin. 24). However, there can be interference in transmission of conducted innate information/F (Prin. 29). Chiropractors are concerned with the normal transmission of innate impulses for coordination of actions (Prin. 31, 32). Our raison d'être is to locate, analyze, and participate in the correction of vertebral subluxations.

When inforuns are transformed they are coded units. If they are centralized in the brain, they are called innate impulses to be conducted through nerves for coordination of activities. If they emanate from the tissue cell, they are called innate rays to be radiated from within the cell to control its components for metabolism. The information/F is now outside the innate realm and in the material realm, in which they can be computed to form instructions and be expressed in physical form (Prin. 13). Chiropractic is concerned exclusively with innate impulses. An innate impulse is more than just a material chemo-electric impulse. It is a chemo-electric impulse with an instructive message affixed to it computed and coded by the innate law for coordination of activities.

Transformation/encoding modifies universal information/F that is potentially deconstructive into constructive innate information/F to maintain the body alive (Prin. 21, 26). The transformation/encoding is in a sense a re-characterization that provides instructions contained within the innate impulse. By analogy, a cellphone in the 1980s, dubbed a brick,[15] was only a phone to make a call without wires. When Apple constructed the iPhone, in January 2007, it was different; the properties and functions of the phone had amplified. It was no longer only a brick, it was the iPhone. A wireless phone was been converted into a portable computer device with a multitude of functions including a camera and locator capability.[16] Transformation/coding is the process by which the innate law computes information/F and modifies it from being ONLY a universal state into a NEW innate state for use in the body and coordination of activities.

ART. 59. THE SEVENTH STEP OF THE NORMAL COMPLETE CYCLE FOR COORDINATION OF ACTIVITIES: INNATE IMPULSE

An innate impulse is a unit of instructive innate information/F for a specific part of the body, for a specific moment, for coordination actions (Prin. 23, 32). It is a special instruction to a body part for the current instant. It differs from universal information/F in that it is constructive for the parts of the body, for a particular moment, for coordination of activities. While universal information/F are not constructive in particular for the living body, they are for all moments generally maintaining everything in existence and are too general to be coordinative (Prin. 10, 14, 15).

It is not fully understood what innate impulses are. This is no reflection on chiropractic, for, even today in 2022, engineers, electricians, computer programmers, and physicists do not really know what an electronic impulse or what electricity is, except to say that it is a form of energy comprised of the flow of electrons.[17] Yet, they know its principles and manifestations and are able to make practical application of this knowledge. Chiropractors know the principles of innate impulses and information/F,

---

15. "The Cellphones of the 1980s." techcentral.co.za/the-cellphones-of-the-1980s/191544 Jan 2015.

16. "Steve Jobs debuts the iPhone." history.com/this-day-in-history/steve-jobs-debuts-the-iphone. Published Aug 2012.

17. Bellis, Mary. "What is Electricity?" thoughtco.com/what-is-electricity-4019643 Sept 2018.

their manifestations, and possibility of interference in their transmission (Prin. 1, 8, 9, 10, 13, 14, 15, 23, 24, 25, 26, 27, 28, 29, 31). They can make practical application of this knowledge to restore the transmission of innate impulses through the location, analysis, and facilitation of the correction of vertebral subluxations. Whatever the innate information/F is, chiropractors have named a unit of it, an impulse. For coordination of activities, an innate impulse and for metabolism of tissue cells, an innate ray/wave. This is done with the same justification that the electrical engineers have named a unit of electrical current an ampere, or that the computer programmers have named a unit of data a bit.

Each body part requires specific innate impulses for coordination of actions every moment (Prin. 23, 32). Since there are multitudes of body parts it takes multitudes of innate impulses for them every moment. There are new ones for every adaptive change. These innate impulses are necessary and vital, for coordination of activities, for the particular moment for which they are characterized by the innate law and no other. They cannot be stored, held, or damned back. If this were possible the innate impulses would immediately become useless. They are the instantiation of the principle of continuous supply and computation (Prin. 33). Going back to our analogy of the iPhone, if a text message with important instructions was delayed due to interference between the tower signal transmissions, there would be consequences in momentum and timing. It is always necessary and vital to have normal transmission of innate impulses (Prin. 27, 29). That is why chiropractors insure there are no vertebral subluxations that interfere with the transmission of innate impulses of the body (Prin. 31).

ART. 60. THE EIGHTH STEP OF THE NORMAL COMPLETE CYCLE FOR COORDINATION OF ACTIVITIES: PROPULSION/CONDUCTIVITY

Propulsion is the initial momentum of innate impulses from the brain cells that will be transmitted through the conductors. It is the act of origin causing the innate impulse to have specific motion in order to be conducted through the nerves.

The term is derived from *propel* to drive forward or onward" by the Merriam-Webster Dictionary. The innate impulse is both non-material (instructive code) and material (chemo-bio-electric carrier, the nerve cell). The innate impulse is information/F that has been adapted and instantiated in the innate field by the innate law. It has then been centralized in the brain to be propelled through nerve conductors (neuron-transmitters) for the coordination of activities (Prin. 28, 32). For example, when one types on the keyboard of a computer, non-material codes in the forms of letters, words, and sentences appear on the screen as instructions to be seen in the material realm. If they are to be printed on a sheet of paper, the key-symbol "print" must be pressed and it provides the initial momentum to propel/conduct the code signals (material and non-material) to be transmitted to the printer. In the same way, the departure of the innate impulse from the brain cell, to be conducted through nerves is the stage of propulsion, its initial momentum.

REVIEW QUESTIONS ARTICLES 51 - 60

1. Is a living tree governed by the innate law of living things?

2. Which kind of living thing can live in a wider range of environment?

3. What is the innate realm?

4. What does the innate law adapt to maintain an organism alive?

5. What is innate control?

6. What is educated control?

7. What is the brain cell with respect to the normal complete cycle?

8. What is innate characterization/re-organizing?

9. Explain the step, transformation/coding.

10. What is innate impulse?

11. Can innate impulse be stored or stockpiled?

12. What is propulsion/conductivity?

ART. 61. THE NINTH STEP OF THE NORMAL COMPLETE CYCLE FOR COORDINATION OF ACTIVITIES: EFFERENT NERVE

An efferent nerve is the conductor of innate impulse from brain cell to tissue cell for coordination of activities. The nerve-tissue cell consists of neurons that communicate within the body by transmitting innate impulses for coordination of actions of ALL the parts of the body (Prin. 23). Neurons have many long cellular dendrites and axons that extend from their central bodies (Fig. 10). Efferent neurons transmit signals called innate impulses from the brain cells to the tissue cells of body parts. Efferent nerves are neuron-transmitters of innate impulses, while the parts of the body are receptors of innate impulses.

Efferent nerves are comprised of tissue cells called neurons with a body, dendrites and axons that act as information-highways to carry innate impulses between the brain, the spinal cord and all the parts of the body. Efferent nerves are one-way neuron-transmitters as they only transmit innate impulses from the brain-CPU to the body part-receptor.

ART. 62. THE TENTH STEP OF THE NORMAL COMPLETE CYCLE FOR COORDINATION OF ACTIVITIES: TRANSMISSION

Transmission, on the efferent side, is the passage of the innate impulse from the brain cell to the tissue cell of a body part. It is the conduction of the innate information/F for coordination of activities (Prin. 23, 28).

The function of the nerve system is to transmit innate impulses and educated impulses from the brain cell to the tissue cell of a body part (efferent), along with its feedback trophic impulses, from the tissue cell of a body part to the brain cell (afferent), which includes the sensory impulses. The innate impulses, for coordination of activities, are coded into instructions and are transmitted on the efferent side to various parts of the body from one neuron to another crossing synapses. The spinal nerves innervate much of the body and connect through the spinal column to the spinal cord. While innate impulses and educated impulses are conveyed by nerve impulse, which is an electro-chemical neuron excitation conducted through the nerve system of the body, the student is cautioned to not confuse the two. The encoded instruction of an innate information/F is purely non-material, non-discrete, hence the term "innate". On the other hand, the nerve impulse is purely material, discrete, hence the term "impulse." An innate impulse is therefore both non-material and material. A multitude of neurons are constructed into nerve fibers by the innate law with a myriad of frequencies to conduct innate impulses, educated impulses, trophic impulses, and sensory impulses. The higher the frequency of conduction, the greater will be the momentum of the transmission. The only way a nerve fiber can interfere with the innate impulse is through a change in the frequency of the impulse conduction. That is precisely the consequence of a vertebral subluxation, which is the condition of a vertebra that has lost its proper juxtaposition with the one above or the one below, or both; to an extent less than a luxation; which impinges nerves and interferes with the transmission of innate impulses (Art. 26). The vertebral subluxation causes a lack of ease at the site of the impingement that alters the frequency of innate impulse conduction, changing the momentum of the transmission, thus violating the principle of coordination (Prin. 29, 30, 31, 32).

ART. 63. THE ELEVENTH STEP OF THE NORMAL CYCLE FOR COORDINATION OF ACTIVITIES: TISSUE CELL

The tissue cell is the smallest unit of tissue considered in function. It is that unit of tissue which with innate information/F will perform one unit of function for coordination of activities. It is a unit of living E/matter. It may have many functions but the one related to the normal complete cycle is the function for which it is constructed to coordinately benefit the welfare of all the other parts of the body (Prin. 32).

The Merriam-Webster Dictionary defines *cells* as:

"A small usually microscopic mass of protoplasm bounded externally by a semi-permeable membrane, usually including one or more nuclei and various other organelles with their products, capable alone or interacting with other cells of performing at the fundamental functions of life, and forming the smallest structural unit of living matter capable of functioning independently."

Tissue is defined as:

"an aggregate of cells usually of a particular kind together with their intercellular substance that form one of the structural materials of a plant or an animal."

In chiropractic, we study the tissue cell physiologically and histologically as other sciences do. In these studies, a tissue cell is the smallest unit of living E/matter. That it is organic E/matter and cellular organisms have signs of life. Because of this, the student will study many biological fields to understand the breath and depth of chiropractic, its impact on the body, and why its objective is pursued.

In chiropractic, we consider the tissues that are dependent on the innate impulse to be instructed for coordination of activities. Chiropractors aim at the correction of vertebral subluxation for the restoration of the transmission of innate impulses for coordination of actions that demonstrate the activity of the organizing principle of the living E/matter of the body (Prin. 20). Chiropractic is interested in the study of E/matter in the sense that it looks continually for the activity of the innate law, namely the innate control for coordination of actions of all the parts of the living body. Therefore, the chiropractic objective is to correct vertebral subluxations to restore the transmission of instructions, contained within the innate impulses, from innate law to the tissue cell, for coordination of activities during its lifespan, while it functions and still has the ability to reproduce itself.

Once again, the chiropractic objective is to remove the impingement (correction of vertebral subluxations) that interferes with the frequency of innate impulse conduction, thereby restoring the momentum of transmission to satisfy the principle of coordination (Prin. 29, 30, 31, 32).

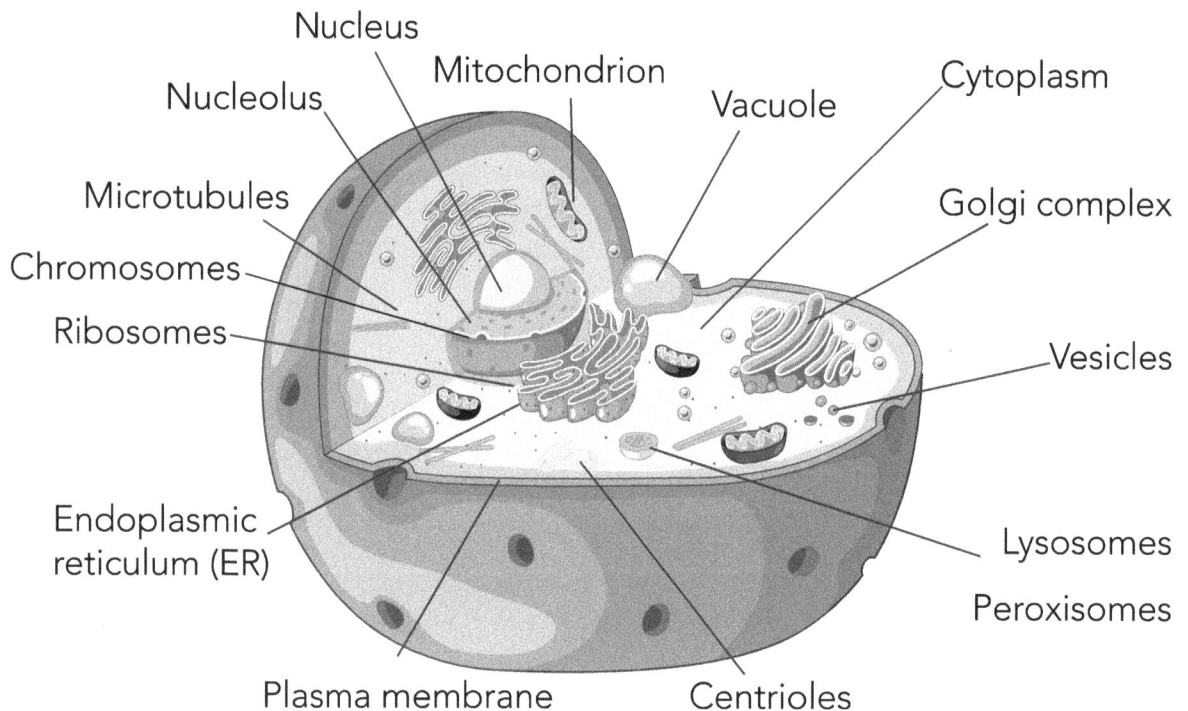

Fig. 11. Shows intra-cell particulates (see lexicon) that are governed by the innate law through innate rays/waves for metabolism of the cell (Art. 27). The basic membrane-bound unit is comprised of the fundamental molecules of life for all living things. A single cell is often a complete organism in itself. Other cells divide, differentiate, and cooperate with other specialized cells forming multi-cellular organisms, such as the body of humans and other animals.

ART. 64. THE SIGNS OF LIFE

Tne Merriam-Webster Dictionary defines *life* as:

1a: The quality that distinguishes a vital and functional being from a dead body.

1b: A principle or force that is considered to underlie the distinctive quality of animate beings.

1c: An organic state characterized by capacity for metabolism, growth, reaction to stimuli, and reproduction.

2: the sequence of physical and mental experiences that make up the existence of an individual

The signs of life are the evidence of organization. Organization is everywhere in the universe and bespeaks intelligence. Therefore the signs of life are the evidence of the intelligence of life. The signs of life are also the evidence of local activity of an innate law controlling and governing the body of a living thing. As mentioned in Art. 50, the innate law of living things is an essential continuous extension of the universal principle of organization designed and programmed by a universal intelligence. Living E/matter expresses innate information/E that maintains it alive for its lifespan according to universal laws (Prin. 13, 21, 24).

There are five primary signs of life: assimilation, excretion, adaptability, growth, and reproduction (Prin. 18). Life is the quality which distinguishes animate E/matter of the vegetable and animal kingdoms from inanimate E/matter of elements of the periodic table that are non-living. Living E/matter has the property of being adaptable to the environment. The signs of life reveal the continual adaptation of universal information/F and living E/matter by the constant local activity of the innate law within the body of living things (Prin. 18, 19, 20). It is the innate control that instructs every tissue cell through innate rays or waves for metabolism and innate impulses for the coordination of activities. The practice of chiropractic is only concerned with the correction of vertebral subluxation for the restoration of the transmission of innate impulses conducted through nerves. Of course, the specific metabolism of each cell at every moment is also dependent upon coordination of actions of all the parts of the body (Prin. 23). Without coordination of action of all the parts, there cannot be proper use for the body, even though there can be metabolism for the cell, which keeps it alive but isolated. However, it is then of no use to the body and will in time, eventually die.

Let's us take a closer look, through the lens of the principles of chiropractic's basic science, and examine the five signs of life in order of importance: assimilation, excretion, adaptability, growth, and reproduction. It must be noted that only one sign needs to be present for E/matter to be living. Of course if an organism manifests any sign, even if it is not completely perceivable, it will also manifest the signs preceding it. For example, if an organism demonstrates excretion, then it must assimilate; if it demonstrates growth, it must be assimilating, excreting, and adapting, and so on.

ART. 65. ASSIMILATION

Assimilation is the 100%/perfect innate ability of an organism to selectively take into its body material nutrients, and make them part of itself according to the innate law as an organized normal software computation program moment to moment (Prin. 33).

The metabolism of each cell of a living thing is controlled by the innate law (Prin. 20, 23). Philosophically, direct your attention to the fact that any living thing that is able to take food materials into its body, takes only that which it is receptive to in its construction, or maintenance. It does not have receptors for materials that cannot be used in that process. This indicates selective ability. Selection requires localized and repeated specific computation, moment-by-moment. Specific computation requires a 100%/perfect program that is a perfectly engineered software by intelligence, which is intrinsic to the body of every living things. It is called the innate law of living things. This innate software is programmed according to specific designs of living E/matter, in order to construct living structures based on genetic materials that are also governed by the innate law (Prin. 21). For human beings, selection of food for assimilation involves the educated brain and the external environment. What human beings put in their body will either be assimilated for use or will be eliminated if it is of no use, all within the limitation of E/matter (Prin. 24).   Once the substance is ingested, the computing of selectivity is an innate function that is programmed to operate only according to universal laws (Prin. 23, 24). This underscores the importance to choose wisely with our educated brain what we ingest and to also make sure that there are no vertebral subluxations that interfere with the transmission of innate impulses.

Assimilation is not only the taking of nutrients, but the utilization of those nutrients by incorporating them as part of the living thing. This is due to a 100%/perfect innate program in accordance with the principle of continuous supply and computation (Prin. 33), designed by a universal intelligence. It involves interoperability amongst different parts of the body including the digestive system.

ART. 66. EXCRETION

Excretion is the 100%/perfect innate ability of an organism to selectively give off waste materials, which are no longer of use in that structure according to the innate law as an organized normal software computation program moment to moment (Prin. 27, 33).

The innate law is controlling the computation of a multitude of functions of physical systems directed toward the selective elimination of materials that have served their purpose and are not usable. If any undesirable materials are in the food that are foreign to the uses of the organism, the 100%/perfect innate law will adapt and compute its information/F content and will sort them out controlling its elimination through the interoperability of all the body parts involved. This elimination will occur mainly through a process of propulsion within the gastrointestinal tract. Waste byproducts of metabolism will be excreted through various forms of elimination of the excretory system (urinating, defecating, sweating, breathing, coughing, sneezing) again through interoperability. All of these physiological functions are controlled and computed by the innate law for the mutual benefit of all the parts of the body according to universal laws (Prin. 23, 24).

ART. 67. ADAPTABILITY

Adaptability is the 100%/perfect innate ability of an organism to interface with information/F that it is subjected to and act on it, for processing, whether universal or innate. All the signs of life are specific motions of subatomic particles of living E/matter. They are manifested by specific motion in E/matter (Prin. 14) otherwise they would not be considered signs of life. Adaptability is the feature of a system's ability to compute and process information/F by way of instantaneously changing moment to moment. Living E/matter is organized and constructed with the capability to be adaptable by the innate law. Living E/matter can be adapted and modified according to internal or external information/F emanating from life circumstances.

The student is cautioned not to confuse adaptability, adaptation and 100%/perfect instantaneous integral adaptation (See lexicon.)

100%/perfect instantaneous integral adaptation is an innate process, which takes place within the innate realm. It is strictly non-material. It is a non-discrete process occurring in the innate field to adapt the interoperability of an organism for use in its body to maintain it alive (Prin. 21, 23). It is integral in the sense that it addresses all the parts of the body as well as all of the universal information/F that needs to be adapted simultaneously.

Adaptation is the physical process that takes place as the manifestation of 100%/perfect instantaneous integral adaptation as the expression of innate rays/waves for metabolism and innate impulses for coordination of activities. It is the physical representation of it.

Adaptability is the ability to perform the above processes. It means that adaptability is the ability of living E/matter to interface with a continuous supply of information/F (Prin. 1, 33), which is from the environment (internal or external). The student's attention is called to the word interface, which indicates an innate act. If the innate law was not intrinsic to the living structure, if there was no innate law it wouldn't be living, and it would receive the information/F without innate action, just like a rock. It would be dead. Organisms, however, show more complex levels of organization that manifest action. In other word, living organisms demonstrate a continuous varying levels of complexity of organization and consequently also of action that indicate an interface with continuous exposure to information/F through their adaptability. This detailed, instantaneous and specific innate adaptation certifies the presence of highly defined organizational states of living E/matter that bespeak intelligent interface. The process of computing information/F, within living E/matter for adaptation, is the function of the 100%/perfect innate law (Prin. 22, 23), which is instantaneously integral and normal (Prin. 27). It bespeaks the perfect design of a 100%/perfectly programmed innate law from a perfect universal intelligence, of unlimited potentials and possibilities for infinite computations at every moment. It is called instantaneous integral adaptation. The manifestation of this instantaneous computation process of integral adaptation may require some time (Prin. 6) because of the limitations of E/matter (Prin. 24).

All organisms have the benefit of instantaneous integral adaptation. If they did not, they could not be alive at all (Prin. 23). An organism that has a more highly developed third sign of life is higher in the scale of life because of its ability to adapt more to environmental conditions and thus extend its range of possible environment. Human beings have the most powerful organ of instantaneous integral adaptation, the educated brain, hence a greater adaptability. They also have higher sensibility and reasoning.

This 100%/perfect instantaneous integral adaptation occurs in the innate field which is non-discrete. The innate field is wherever the innate law is active within the body of the living thing. It is a 100%/perfect system of structural operation of living E/matter with instantaneous interoperability according to universal laws (Prin. 22, 23, 24).

ART. 68. GROWTH

Growth is the 100%/perfect innate ability of an organism to expand to mature size according to a 100%/perfect innate program and is dependent upon the ability of assimilation. What was said about an organized systematic programmable process in regards to assimilation and excretion also applies to instantaneous integral processes in growth. There is plenty of evidence of 100%/perfect innate control shown in growth. To perfectly grow an organism to mature size requires a 100%/perfect innate software program, designed by intelligence to compute all the information/F into instructions providing properties and actions to living E/matter. Instructive information/F will expand living E/matter within exact and specific proportions. A tissue cell or any other organism of a given kind is the same around the world. There is an innate control related to size and direction. Living things do not grow beyond their mature size, which is under direct control of the intrinsic innate law of living things according to universal laws (Prin. 20, 22, 23, 24). Growth is a permanent irreversible process. All living things grow, whereas non-living things do not grow.

ART. 69. REPRODUCTION

Reproduction is the 100%/perfect innate ability of a living thing to produce offspring. It is the exclusive capability of living E/matter to perpetuate. This sign of life, as the others demonstrates organization that bespeaks intelligence. An organism's affinity to reproduce shows 100%/perfect integral innate processing of limitless possibilities and potentials. There is always an innate control manifested in all forms of reproduction to preserve an organized balance. When an organism produces an offspring, it perpetuates its kind. If this were not true, its kind would not continue.

In the body, the instruction of the innate law does not grant all cells to reproduce their type extemporaneously. It they did, it would not be coordinated action and it would not preserve the size, shape, and functions of the body. When there is an uncontrolled replication of cells in the body, it results in ineffectuality of use in the body.

In the study of these signs of life, the expression "100%/perfect innate ability" is mentioned frequently. We are directly referring to the organization of the living thing, which bespeaks non-discrete intelligence. The student is reminded that we use the word organization and 100%/perfect innate ability synonymously regarding living E/matter. The student may wonder why motor function is not named as one of the signs of life, since the most obvious sign is motion. It is worth noting that all five signs of life are motion and therefore, it is unnecessary to name motion as sign (Prin. 18). The peculiarity of this motion, however, distinguishes it from other observable motion (Prin. 14, 15), in that it is adaptive according to universal laws (Prin. 24). This motion demonstrates a 100%/perfect innate program of computations of limitless potentials and possibilities that again bespeaks intelligence. None of these are shown in the motion of non-living E/matter, like a rolling rock.

The student is cautioned not to confuse the signs of life of excretion and reproduction with the primary functions of elimination and replication. There is some difference and it will be explained later in volume three.

ART. 70. DUPLICATION OF CELLS

The duplication of cells concerns the expansion of cells in the developmental or embryonic centers which are derived from the blastoderm. It is a process by which cells replicate their contents and then divide to yield two cells with similar contents. In chiropractic, duplication is considered a center that is composed of cells, representing one of the four forms of primary tissues. There is a center for each kind of primary tissues, so that all kinds of cells may be duplicated for growth, daily maintenance and reparation. The continuity of life from one cell to another is due to what is called the cell cycle, which is an organized sequence of stages of the life of a cell. It is also called cellular replacement.

Duplication is very closely associated with the growth, reparation, and maintenance of a cell. Considering duplication as a function, our study can be made more exact as we examine a tissue cell as a functional unit. In order that the body may grow, it must have more cells, and this is accomplished by the duplication of tissue cells whose function is to serve that purpose.

In the body, these duplicative cells are in the reproductive centers, as, the embryonic or developmental centers derived from the blastoderm, which is the primitive membrane of cell that results from the subdivision of the fertilized egg. This process is the result of the functioning of the expansion centers in generative organs of the parents, which is always under the control of the innate law within the limits of adaptation (Prin. 24). The purpose of these special cells is replicative function, one of the nine primary functions.

One of the most fundamental events of life is cell division, which is dependent on a parent cell increasing its intracellular content, dispensing it, and duplicating its genetic material. It is the reconstruction in exact duplicate of a cell with identical genetic instructive information. This process is continuous throughout the life of the living thing and is know as the cell cycle.

Cell division is called mitosis. Its objective is to divide the chromatin (material of the chromosomes) into two identical arrangements and enclose each portion in a nucleus. In chiropractic, the cause of mitosis is explained by the theory of cell expansion. It states that from the time of fertilization of the ovum, the possibilities and potentials of all the cells of the body, which are to be used in the development and in the maintenance of its structure, are contained in that one cell.

These possibilities and potentialities are expanded to full grown cells as provided by computed and coded instructive information/F of the innate law for constructing and repairing purposes. This action manifests as mitosis. We can observe the cell division but cannot see the unexpanded cells. However, this does not weaken the theory of the cell expansion since the theory is based upon results rather than upon what can be observed. The student should keep in mind that there is infinity in smallness as well as magnitude. It is not possible to see all that happens in a tissue cell. Chiropractic is about what is possible according to universal laws (Prin. 24).

In the normal body, cells are not duplicated faster than what is required for growth, reparation, and propagation of species. If they do, through a lack innate control, there will be ineffectuality of use in the body and/or in-coordination of action of the parts of the body.

Some cells are never innately programmed to duplicate; certain other cells are but only at such times and in the manner in which they are innately programmed. For example muscles cells replicated from developmental centers but at certain times, as in case of a wound, computation of innate information/F by the innate law will cause connective tissue to proliferate.

Note: Reproduction as a sign of life refers to the propagation of species of the whole unit. It is the propagation of a specific type of organism.

 Replication as a primary function refers to the functioning of an organ whose purpose is duplication as a coordinative act, from the developmental centers, to be used for growth and reparation. The expansion centers are of all kinds of tissue, since all kinds of tissue are necessary in growth and reparation according to the 100%/perfect innate program controlling each particular part of the body of the living thing. It calls attention to the necessity for normal transmission of innate impulses.

REVIEW QUESTIONS FOR ARTICLES 61 - 70

1. What is efferent nerve?

2. Explain transmission.

3. What tissue is used for transmission?

4. What are signs of life?

5. How may we know the perfection of organization by the signs of life?

6. What is assimilation?

7. What is excretion?

8. What is adaptability?

9. Differentiate between adaptability, adaptation, and 100%/perfect instantaneous integral adaptation?

10. What is growth?

11. What is reproduction?

12. What is duplication of cell?

13. What is replication?

14. Differentiate between reproduction as a sign of life and replication as a primary function.

15. What is the theory of cell expansion in chiropractic?

At this time, the interjection of some anatomy and physiology of reproduction will reveal the intelligent design and continuous innate control that adapts and organizes the living body through a 100%/perfect innate program of unlimited capabilities (Prin. 20, 21, 23). This 100%/perfect innate program continually computes, moment by moment, all possibilities and potentialities of all the cells of the body according to universal laws (Prin. 23, 24, 33). Reproduction of one's own kind through gene transfer from parent to offspring reveals, philosophically with certitude, organization due to a 100%/perfect innate law that is designed and programmed by intelligence.

ART. 71. THE SPERMATOZOON

Spermatozoon [sper″mah-to-zo′on] (pl. spermatozo′a) (Gr.) :

A mature male germ cell, the specific output of the testes, which fertilizes the mature ovum (secondary oocyte) in sexual reproduction. It is microscopic in size, looks like a translucent tadpole, and has a flat elliptical head containing a spherical center section, and a long tail by which it propels itself with a vigorous lashing movement. Spermatozoa are produced in the seminiferous tubules of the testes. The developmental stages of the germ cell are the spermatogonium, spermatocyte, spermatid, and finally spermatozoon. When mature, the spermatozoa are carried in the semen. At the climax of coitus, the semen is discharged into the vagina of the female. A single discharge (about a teaspoonful of semen on the average) may contain more than 250 million spermatozoa. Only a few of these will travel as far as the fallopian tubes; if an ovum is present there, and if the head of a single sperm penetrates the ovum, fertilization takes place. adj., adj spermatozo′al.

The spermatozoon is controlled by the innate law through instructive innate information/F constructed into innate rays/waves that emanate from the cell itself, carrying possibilities and potentialities to be fleshed out from the male for the reproduction of the species.[18]

Even though, the practice of chiropractic is concerned only with innate impulses that are conducted through nerves according to the principles of its basic science, it is chiropractic philosophy that explains the intelligent design and programming of an organizing principle. Since organization bespeaks intelligence, the cause of this intelligent 100%/perfect universal principle of organization, including its essential continuation as the innate law of living things, stems from a universal intelligence. The continuous action of intelligence through multiple complex levels and states of organization of E/matter, spanning the broadest outlook from divided to condensed E/matter and on to adaptive living E/matter.

ART. 72. THE OVUM

Ovum [o′vum] (pl. *o′va*) (L.) :

The female reproductive or germ CELL which after fertilization is capable of developing into a new member of the same species; called also **egg**. The term is sometimes applied to any stage of the fertilized germ cell during cleavage and even until hatching or birth of the new individual. The human ovum consists of protoplasm that contains some yolk, enclosed by a cell wall consisting of two layers, an outer one (ZONAPELLUCIDA) and an inner thin one (**vitelline** MEMBRANE). There is a large nucleus (germinal vesicle) within which is a nucleolus (germinal spot)[19]

The ovum is controlled by the innate law through instructive innate information/F, that are innate rays/waves, emanating from within the cell itself carrying possibilities and potentialities to be fleshed out from the female for the reproduction of the species. When the ovum is successfully penetrated by the spermatozoon these mingled possibilities and potentialities represent the sum total of all the adaptations of the parent cells that have effectively related to environmental experiences and have developed accordingly.

---

18. MillerKeane Encyclopedia and Dictionary of Medicine, Nursing, and Allied Health. Seventh Edition. Saunder, and imprint of Elsiver, Inc. 2003 p. 1652

19. MillerKeane Encyclopedia and Dictionary of Medicine, Nursing, and Allied Health. p.1277

ART. 73. THE PRONUCLEUS

Pronucleus [pro-noo´kle-us]: The haploid nucleus of a germ cell.

The female pronucleus the haploid nucleus of the fully mature oocyte, which loses its nuclear envelope and liberates its chromosomes to meet the synapsis with those from the male pronucleus.

In the male pronucleus the nuclear material of the head of a spermatozoon, after it has penetrated the oocyte and acquired a pronuclear membrane.[20]

The ovum is a single cell which when it is fertilized contains chromatin from both parents, by means of which the genetic characteristic of both male and female is transmitted to the offspring. In the process of fertilization the head of the spermatozoon penetrates the ovum, leaving its flagellum to drop off and be absorbed. The ovum has two nuclei, one of its own and one that came with the spermatozoon. These two centrosomes then act as a basis for the first cleavage or cell division. As cell division begins, the two centrosomes move to opposite ends of the cell helping to separate the replicated chromosomes. This single ovum with its two nuclei is then ready for immediate development under the innate control of the innate law, a process demonstrating intelligent computations within the fertilized ovum from the instructions of innate rays/waves.

ART. 74. MULBERRY MASS OR MORULA.

Morula [mor´ulah]: solid mass of cells (**BLASTOMERES**) resembling a mulberry, formed by cleavage of a **ZYGOTE** (fertilized ovum).

The solid mass of blastomeres resulting from the early cleavage divisions of the zygote.

In oocytes with little yolk, the morula is a spheroid mass of cells; in forms with considerable yolk, the configuration of the morula stage is greatly modified.

It is the spherical embryonic mass of blastomeres formed before the blastula and resulting from cleavage of the fertilized ovum.[21]

In the few hours following the fertilization of the ovum, the cell has divided into many other cells by mitosis, forming a solid mass of cells resembling a mulberry with its little globules. This is the early stage in the embryonic development. The cells of the morula continue to replicate themselves it travels to the uterus where it becomes stationary upon a spot of its surface. All of these multiples of possibilities and of potentialities are computed and processed through the innate control of the innate law. It demonstrates 100%/perfect intelligent innate software program within the morula expressing instructive innate information/F that emanates from innate rays/waves (Prin. 13).

---

20. MillerKeane Encyclopedia and Dictionary of Medicine, Nursing, and Allied Health. p. 1451

21. MillerKeane Encyclopedia and Dictionary of Medicine, Nursing, and Allied Health. p. 1145

ART. 75. THE PRIMITIVE STREAK OR TRACE

Primitive streak: a faint white trace at the caudal end of the embryonic disk, formed by movement of cells at the onset of mesoderm formation, providing the first evidence of the embryonic axis. It eventually undergoes degenerative changes and disappears.

It is the ridge of epiblast in the midline at the caudal end of the embryonic disc from which arises the intraembryonic mesoderm and definitive endoderm; achieved by inward and then lateral migration of cells; in human embryos, it appears on day 15 and provides visual evidence of the cephalocaudal axis. An ectodermal ridge in the midline at the caudal end of the embryonic disc from which arises the intraembryonic mesoderm; achieved by inward and then lateral migration of cells; in human embryos, it appears on day 15 and gives a cephalocaudal axis to the developing embryo.[22]

In the course of a very short time a dark line appears on the surface of the mulberry mass; it has a knob on the anterior end. This dark streak with the knob is the spinal cord and brain. It is the first recognizable structure to appear. It stays on the surface for a short time and then sinks slowly into the mulberry mass as the layers are formed. This intelligent construction and development of the embryo is expressing instructive innate information/F that emanates from innate rays/waves (Prin. 13). It demonstrates intelligent computation under the perfect innate control of the innate law of living things (Prin. 23).

ART. 76. THE BLASTODERM

Blastoderm: disk of cells lying between the yolk sac and the amniotic cavity, from which the embryo develops.

The thin, discshaped cell mass of a young embryo and its extraembryonic extensions over the surface of the yolk; when fully formed, all three primary germ layers (ectoderm, endoderm, and mesoderm) are present.[23]

In the blastoderm the cells are arranged in three layers from the instructive information/F of the innate law. These three layers are the germinal cells from which the tissues of the body are developed. They are ectoderm, endoderm, and mesoderm.

ART. 77. THE THREE LAYERS OF THE BLASTODERM

From the outer layer, the ectoderm, the skin and nerve tissues are developed. The middle layer, the mesoderm, develops into the tissues that make up the bulk of the body. The inner layer, the endoderm, develops into the tissues that make up the mucous linings of the inner organs of the body. From these three layers, the four primary tissues of the body are derived.

As the blastoderm becomes the body, the germinal cells of its three layers become the expansive centers of the body in which cells are expanded for the purpose of growth and reparation. The innate control actually maintains throughout as an organized group whose purpose it is to replicate cells. They replicate not only their own kind, but there are germs that duplicate cells that carry forth all cell possibilities and potentialities to the next generation. The purpose of the latter germinal cells is a primary function, called

---

22. MillerKeane Encyclopedia and Dictionary of Medicine, Nursing, and Allied Health. p. 1684

23. MillerKeane Encyclopedia and Dictionary of Medicine, Nursing, and Allied Health. p. 220

replicative function, for their work is to benefit the body as a whole, which reveals organization from the instructive information/F of the innate law that bespeaks intelligence.

ART. 78. THE FOUR PRIMARY TISSUES

The four primary tissues derived from the three layers of the germinal cells of the blastoderm are: epithelium, muscular, connective, and nerve.

The study of these tissues is included so the student will not fail to notice the structure and capabilities of each form of these primary tissues. Note the characteristic structures of those primary tissues, that are adapted by the innate law from its 100%/perfect programming, according to their roles and purposes which accounts for their presence in the body. When motor function is necessary to meet environmental requirements (internal or external), the innate law will generate instruction that will compute and process specific information/F to be expressed by E/matter manifesting the motion of a soft, elongated elastic muscle cell with a moveable protoplasm (Prin. 13, 14, 15). When environmental requirements necessitate a framework to support the body, the innate control will compute specific information/F that will manifest the motion of some hard "rock-like" bone cells, capable of passive resistance. The 100%/perfect programming of the innate law can compute, process, code, and adapts infinite possibilities and potentialities of information/F and E/matter necessary to interact to the internal and external environment of the body moment to moment according to universal laws (Prin. 22, 23, 24). The body of a living thing is truly a living computer that is controlled by a 100%/perfect innate software capable of computing, processing and adapting infinite possibilities and potentialities to keep the body alive (Prin. 21). The 100%/perfect software of the body is the innate law of living things (Prin. 33). It is an innate law, with unlimited instructive information/F that controls the body of a living thing according to universal laws (Prin. 20). Being 100%/perfect, it is absolute and limitless. It does not err and acts only if it is possible according to universal laws. The instructions of innate law are always normal and within the limits of adaptation (Prin. 24, 27).

ART. 79. THE TWELFTH STEP OF THE NORMAL COMPLETE CYCLE FOR COORDINATION OF ACTIVITIES: RECEPTION

 Reception is the arrival of the innate impulse at the body part (receptor) for coordination of actions of that part which is interoperable with other body parts. It is the receiving of the innate code containing a specific instructive information/F for coordination of activities. It is the receipt of an instructive coded input message computed by the innate law.

When a tissue cell of a body part is safe and sound, it is in a wholesome state of construction, robust and alert, ready to receive normally (Prin. 27). From that state, it can immediately act adaptively to the innate impulse (see signs of life). It is able to be receptive of the instructive information/F of the innate law and act accordingly in a normal way (Prin. 27). It has good and normal expression (Prin. 13). For the tissue cell to express the innate information/F normally it must have safe and sound metabolism, it must be supplied innate rays/waves and nutrients necessary for its fitness. On the other hand, if the tissue cell of a body part is not expressing the innate instruction effectively, or is injured or is poisoned, it cannot be receptive or act efficiently. When the tissue cell of a body part is not at its best, it is in a lower state of organization than it should be and its adaptive action will always be proportionate to its state of organization. Even after perfect transmission of innate impulse has been restored it will require some time for the body part to be brought back to its proper state through cellular replication, therefore the element of time enters (Prin. 6).

It demonstrates that the innate law will adapt information/F and E/matter for the body only if it is possible according to universal laws (Prin. 24). For example, suppose there is a vertebral subluxation that is interfering with the transmission of the innate impulses which is violating the principle of coordination (Prin. 5, 24, 29, 31, 32). This cause of in-coordination of actions of some part of the body elsewhere may affect an imbalance of body chemistry in quality or quantity that will then hinder soundness of tissue cells of some other part of the body somewhere else. This could compromise its innate-normal activity. This underscores the importance of practicing the chiropractic objective, which is concluded from the 33 principles of chiropractic's basic science. The chiropractic objective is the location, analysis, and facilitation of the correction of vertebral subluxations for the normal transmission of innate impulses of the body. It is nothing less. It is nothing more. It is nothing else.

Remember that we are studying the normal complete cycle for coordination of activities and that the vertebral subluxation is the uniquely chiropractic entity as a cause of interference to the transmission of innate impulse (Prin. 29, 31). There are other conditions that may occur somewhere else in the body (e.g. a fracture, a dislocation, a prolapsed organ, a tumor, scar tissue, or any other traumatic injury) that can also interfere with the transmission of innate impulses and prompt in-coordination of activities. Chiropractic addresses exclusively the vertebral subluxation causing interference in transmission of innate impulses.

ART. 80. THE THIRTEENTH STEP OF THE NORMAL COMPLETE CYCLE FOR COORDINATION OF ACTIVITIES: PHYSICAL REPRESENTATION

Physical representation is the non-material expressed by the material (Prin. 13). First the non-material coded instruction is decoded by the innate control within the cell. It is then physically manifested as specific motion by the tissue cell (Prin. 14, 15). It is a material form of an innate computation with an instructive purpose. It is the exact manifestation of all the possibilities and potentialities of the moment according to universal laws.

When the innate law adapts information/F and E/matter, the necessary computations are entirely non-discrete and yet, they are real for that specific process. As evidence to our educated abilities, they must be expressed. Every bit of non-discrete information/F within the universe must be expressed by E/matter (Prin. 10, 13, 14, 15). We could not be aware of motion unless we perceive or observe E/matter moving. When we observe or perceive E/matter moving, we must know, if we reason, that either the universal principle of organization or its essential continuation which is the innate law of living things, or both, organized the information/F that set E/matter in motion (Prin. 14, 15, 23). We know that a principle has organized information/F, because the motions are always according to universal laws, either precise unchangeable laws, or the laws of precise instantaneous change-adaptation of the moment. Present motion then is the physical expression of the innate realm of organization bespeaking intelligence, and structures of E/matter are constructions becoming physical representations of innate computation that have been and that are now manifested as observed motions (Prin. 15).

For example, an architect imagines an innovative building. To the architect, the building is real, but it will exist only to him and not to anyone else until the finished edifice portrays what the architect had imagined. A planned or programmed event, a party is but an imagined possibility that will be a physical manifestation (representation) of the planned or programmed possibility when it takes place.

How would anyone know your intentions if you did not express them through material media through speaking, writing, emails or texts? In the same manner, the more elaborate innate computations and coding of infinite possibilities and potentialities of the moment are expressed through the material of every tissue cell of the body parts. The innate law of living things is a 100%/perfect and normal software that is always exact for the moment, every moment in the entire life process of the living thing.

REVIEW QUESTIONS FOR ARTICLES 71 – 80

1. Describe the spermatozoon.

2. Describe an ovum.

3. Describe the pronucleus and how it develops.

4. What is the mulberry mass?

5. What is the primitive streak?

6. What important significance does the primitive streak has?

7. What is a blastoderm?

8. Describe the layers of the blastoderm.

9. Name the four primary tissues and give their origins.

10. What is reception, the 12th step of the cycle?

11. Explain physical representation.

12. Demonstrate intelligent and continuous innate control from one of the above questions.

ART. 81. THE FOURTEENTH STEP OF THE NORMAL COMPLETE CYCLE FOR COORDINATION OF ACTIVITIES: EXPRESSION

Expression is the activity of E/matter, which reveals the manifestation of instructive information/F organized by the innate control, which bespeaks intelligence (Prin. 13, 18). It is a demonstration of manifestation of organized motion (Prin. 14, 15). It indicates 100%/perfect instantaneous integral adaptation from the innate law.

Expression is an output process. It is an act that is detectable through the manifestation of specific motions. It is something becoming evident. This something is the instructive information/F of the innate law as innate impulses with regard to the normal complete cycle for coordination of activities. The manner of its output is very important and significant because the momentum and direction of instructive information/F is computed under innate control and is determined by the quality of the structure of the transmitters or the character and soundness of the instrument of expression (the body part) for its particular role and purpose for coordination of activities. It must be noted that information/F can also be in the form of innate rays or innate waves with regard to other cycles, like the cycle of cell metabolism for example. The study of the purposes of these instruments of expression is the study of function for use in the body with coordinated actions (Prin. 18, 23). In chiropractic, the study of function for use in the body is simply to reveal 100%/perfect innate control within the normal complete cycle according to universal laws. The practice of chiropractic is not concerned with the specific function of body parts. In applying the principles of chiropractic's basic science, the practice of chiropractic is exclusively concerned with the correction of vertebral subluxation to restore the transmission of innate impulses.

ART. 82. THE FIFTEENTH STEP OF THE NORMAL COMPLETE CYCLE FOR COORDINATION OF ACTIVITIES: FUNCTION

Function is the purpose of a tissue cell for use in the body. It has reference to the purpose of a unit of E/matter. As expression reveals the innate control, so function reveals the task-work of a tissue cell. The function of a tissue cell is always according to the character of its structure for use in the body and is the coordinative benefit of all the parts of the body (Prin. 13, 23, 24).

Function is the fulfillment of a purpose, the purpose being the reason for the existence of anything. Everything in existence has reason for existing. The fulfillment of that purpose is function since fulfillment is action. Hence, everything has function and depends upon the character of the structural organization of the instrument of expression. For example, the function of an envelope is to be used to enclose a letter and could not be used for actually writing words on a letter. The function of a pencil is to be used for writing and could not be used to envelope a letter. The function of the lung is to be used as an organ of respiration and could not be used as an organ of sight. Everything has its own function, and that function is what a thing is structurally organized to do, and it accounts for its existence.

A thing may have more than one function or may have a different function at a different time. Some things have multiple functions. Thus, a chair may be used for sitting, as a footstool, standing upon, or as an improvised table. The liver is said to have as many as 500 functions, the major ones are filtration, digestion, metabolism, detoxification, protein synthesis, storage of vitamins, storage of minerals. Regarding the body of a living thing, it is the innate law that controls and governs all the function of all the parts of that particular body in order to maintain it alive (Prin. 20, 21). For this reason chiropractic is concerned exclusively with the correction of vertebral subluxations for the restoration of transmission of innate impulses. Chiropractic ensures that the innate impulses get to their destination without interference from vertebral subluxations.

ART. 83. PRIMARY FUNCTION

A primary function is the purpose of a specific body part's cell for coordination of activities. It is the activity of tissue cells of body parts for the coordinative and mutual benefit of all the parts of the body (Prin. 23). The characteristic structure of a cell of a body part is always in accordance with its primary function, which is for coordination of activities. A tissue cell may have many different motions but only those for coordination are primary. It may fulfill its purpose with no perceptible movement, such as a bone cell.

In the previous article, it was pointed out that a chair might be used for a number of things but it is obvious that the primary function of the chair is to be used for sitting. While it might be used for other things, its coherent use for the aesthetically consistent relationship of the parts, in the household, is strictly the primary function of the chair.

Most parts of the body have more that one purpose. For example, the skin serves as a covering for the body, and also plays a role in secretion, excretion, respiration, radiation, and sensation. All of these are primary functions of the skin. In the normal complete cycle for coordination of activities, however, following our deductive system, we have narrowed our study down to the reception of innate impulses by the tissue cells of body parts. As we go down from the general to the specific, it is evident that the study of function will be the primary purpose of any tissue cell of any body part. This will reveal the continuous innate control of any single cell of the body. This innate control is governed by the innate law, the function of which is using the innate field as an operating system for adapting information/F and E/matter for use in the body so that all body parts of the body will have coordinated action for mutual benefit (Prin. 23). Since there can be interference with conducted innate information/F, which is due to vertebral subluxations (Prin. 29, 31). Chiropractic is only concerned with the correction of vertebral subluxations to restore transmission of innate impulses.

There are four primary tissues in the body, and these four classes are subdivided into other kinds, and these kinds are constructed into a variety of structures. Yet, there is a reason for so many different kinds of structures, for there are many possibilities and potentialities inside and outside the body to be computed for adaptation moment to moment.

An examination of some of these structures reveals that muscle cells, for example, are made to produce movement for the benefit of the whole body, bone cells to offer framework, ligament cells to serve as attachments, epithelial cells to serve as lining and covering, nerve cells to conduct or transmit, and glandular cells to secrete. While all these cells have other motions and purposes than those mentioned, these other motions are for the cell itself, its metabolism, as the signs of the life of the cell (Prin. 18).

Certain classes of these cells are so important in the systems of the body, that when they malfunction they cause more difficulties than others. The level of organization of some cells of certain body parts are more susceptible to difficulties with coordination of their activities than others when there is interference with transmission of innate impulses. We observe that about nine of the primary functions are more susceptible than others to difficulties. They are known in chiropractic as the nine primary functions. Not that these are all the primary functions, but that they are the nine cardinal ones that are more easily observed to lack coordination cause by interference in transmission of innate impulses.

This information simply reveals that the output of expression of living E/matter is dependent on normal transmission of innate impulses for coordination of activities. It is not relevant to the practice of the chiropractic objective which aims only to correct vertebral subluxations for the restoration of transmission of innate impulses, regardless of effects. Chiropractic exclusively addresses the cause of interference in transmission of innate impulses called vertebral subluxation. Chiropractic does not address the effects that are caused by interference in transmission of innate impulses (Prin. 29, 30, 31, 32, 33). Chiropractic is only about cause.

ART. 84. THE NINE PRIMARY FUNCTIONS

Interestingly, the primary functions, which are most commonly involved in in-coordination of actions of the body parts, are approximately nine in number. This is an arbitrary number just to easily demonstrate that the output of expression of living E/matter is affected through a change in its motion.

Here is the list of the nine primary functions:

1. Motor

2. Nutritive

3. Eliminative

4. Caloric

5. Sensory

6. Secretory

7. Reparatory

8. Expansive

9. Replicative

The quality of functions is an output of expression of living E/matter. It is under full control of the innate law. Therefore, it is important that there be no interference in transmission of innate impulses caused by vertebral subluxations.

ART. 85. THE SIXTEENTH STEP OF THE NORMAL COMPLETE CYCLE FOR COORDINATION OF ACTIVITIES: COORDINATION

Coordination is the coherent cooperative action of the parts of the body, controlled and synchronized by the instructive information/F of the innate law. It is the 100%/perfect coherence of purposes of all the structural elements of the body for mutual benefit. It is the 100%/perfect interoperability of all the parts of the body for its welfare as a unit (Prin. 23, 32).

The principle of coordination (Prin. 32) is one of the most fundamental principles of chiropractic's basic science. The integrity of this principle is the "raison d'être" of chiropractic. Everything chiropractic is based on the integrity of the principle of coordination. The fact that a body part is in the body at all, is ample proof that its existence has a purpose (Art. 82). Each tissue cell of a body part is an organism and as such, it has all the possibilities and the potentialities of adaptability governed by the innate control according to universal laws (Prin. 20, 23, 24). It is absolutely essential that the units comprising the body part be this adaptable nature, otherwise the innate law could not control and govern them. If it were not necessary for these units to be adaptable then the innate computation and coding would not be possible since these units would then be comprised of non-living E/matter (Prin. 16, 18).

Coordination is the final step of the efferent side of the cycle and it comes before the first step of the afferent side of the cycle. Coordination is a major principle concerning the practice of the chiropractic objective. It is the principle of coordination that is violated when there is interference in transmission of innate impulses (Prin. 29, 31, 32). The purpose of each tissue cell of the body is for the use and coordinative actions for mutual benefit of all the parts of the body (Prin. 23). It is due to the 100%/perfect innate control adapting, computing, and coding information/F for all possibilities and potentialities of the moment according to universal laws (Prin. 24). It is demonstrated through the output expression of a body part as one of the nine primary functions.

Note: The normal complete cycle for coordination of activities really has no beginning and no end, except that which we ascribe to it. It continually runs and is congruent with the initial principle of chiropractic's basic science (Prin. 1).

ART. 86. THE FIRST AFFERENT STEP OF THE NORMAL COMPLETE CYCLE FOR COORDINATION OF ACTIVITIES: TISSUE CELL

This is the same tissue cell as in step eleven in the efferent side of the cycle. It is the first step on the afferent side of the cycle. Remember, that the tissue cell is the smallest unit of tissue considered in function. It is that unit of tissue, which with one innate impulse will perform one unit of function for coordination of activities. It is a unit of living E/matter. Here, the tissue cell is a receptor that has now received an innate impulse. It is the smallest component of a body part, and it is acting according to its instruction for coordination of activities. It is the material that is manifesting the output from the instruction of an innate impulse and is relating to its internal and external environment through its adaptability. The tissue cell must be safe and sound (in metabolism) to manifest precisely the instruction of innate impulses (Prin. 6, 24).

In chiropractic, the tissue cell is the smallest unit of material, with which one unit of innate information/F expresses one unit of function as it relates to its internal and external environment through its adaptability. All these factors enter into what it does. If sound and safe, the tissue cell will coordinately manifest exactly the coded instruction that it receives as a receptor within its limitations (Prin. 6, 24), as long as there is no interference in transmission of innate impulses of course.

It must be noted that the normal complete cycle for coordination of activities reveals an intrinsic bio-cybernetic feedback loop system, that is under 100%/perfect innate control, allowing for the governing of the interoperability of all body parts by the innate law for coordination of actions (Prin. 32).

ART. 87. THE SECOND AFFERENT STEP OF THE NORMAL COMPLETE CYCLE FOR COORDINATION OF ACTIVITIES: VIBRATION

Vibration is the motion of a tissue cell in performing its function. It is the "raison d'être" of the cell, its life purpose. Tissue cells may be said to have three kinds of motion, namely, functional, metabolic, and physical. The functional is its movement in coordinating its primary function. The metabolic is its movement in the cell manifesting its soundness expressing its signs of life. It is the adapted E/matter by the innate law to maintain it alive. The physical function is its molecular movement, which all E/matter manifests since it is maintained in existence by the universal principle of organization, whether it is in the body of a living thing or as non-living E/matter outside the body. The mere fact that the cell exists, it must manifest physical motion, molecular and atomic movements (Prin. 14). Principle 20 states: A LIVING THING HAS AN INBORN ORGANIZING PRINCIPLE GOVERNING ITS BODY, CALLED THE INNATE LAW OF LIVING THINGS. Inborn, in this case, means intrinsic to all the cells of the body of the living thing. Therefore, the innate control is about every cell of the body.

The functional and metabolic motions of a tissue cell have the characteristics of being adaptive due to the innate law that is intrinsic to their nature. In order to have perfect functional and metabolic vibrations, the tissue cell must be safe and sound (Prin. 6, 24).

Since all E/matter has physical motion (Prin. 14), it is clear that the innate law cannot break a universal law (Prin. 24), yet it can adapt E/matter for use in the body. This is mentioned since bone, a hard rock-like material does not move its living cells when it functions as does muscle. Bone function, which is support, depends upon its hardness and resistive strength. Hardness and resistance are physical properties of E/matter, as a result of coherence, valence, atomic weight. In the body physical properties are adapted and controlled by the innate law. Thus we know that the function of bone depends upon governed physical properties and that these are adapted and supplied to E/matter by an organizing principle (Prin. 1, 20). Coherence and valence are information/F expressed by atoms and molecules, revealing motion at unlimited levels of organization. Therefore, a material of the body, which seemingly has a passive function, is really dependent upon functional motions for coordination of activities through innate impulses, and through innate rays or waves for its metabolic motions. Those innate rays or waves are adapted innate information/F from the innate law and are radiated or oscillated under the innate control intrinsic to every tissue cell. Therefore, there is a metabolic motion within each cell that is governed by the innate control within each cell to sustain its life, according to universal laws (Prin. 20, 21, 23, 24). It is the functional motion of the cell that is used for coordination of activities. When the cell has lost its coordinative ability due to vertebral subluxations, there is still metabolic motion that keeps the cell alive, according to its limitations. When the cell loses its metabolic motion, then the cell retains its physical (atomic and molecular) motion and is no longer living, it is dead. It is deconstructed to its basic elements that are continually maintained in existence by the universal principle of organization. The motion of any tissue of the body is the result of organized information/F by the universal principle of organization (Prin. 1, 13, 14, 15).

This underscores the necessity of the continuous bio-cybernetic feedback loop system of the cycle. Both efferent (input) and afferent (output) sides transmit coded instructive information/F for the coordination of activities of all the parts of the body for mutual benefit (Prin. 23, 28, 32). Even with interference in transmission of innate impulse, the innate law will adapt the tissue cell to keep its metabolic motion so it can be maintained alive. This is why cells continue to be maintained alive even though their functional motion may be altered due to vertebral subluxations. The innate rays or waves are still being organized within the innate field of the cell by the innate law.

The functional motion of a tissue cell constructed within a body part (organ, gland, muscle, etc.) is the movement in coordinating its primary function for the benefit of the whole body. The reason for this is that the primary function of the cell may be to output specific substances that would be required for the metabolic functions of many other tissue cells anywhere in the body. For example, the primary function of the tissue cells of the pituitary gland is to release hormones that will be useful to tissue cells responsible for blood pressure, heart rate, respiration, body temperature, and digestion, just to name a few. For primary functions to be carried out (output) coordinately, the metabolic soundness of the tissue cell is paramount. Hence, we observe the essential necessity of innate rays or waves to be organized in the innate field and radiated or oscillated from within the tissue cell to express metabolic motion within its limitations (Prin. 14, 15, 23, 24). Without sound metabolic motion, the tissue cell cannot carry out its functional motion. This means that it would be possible for the body to have normal transmission of innate impulses (no vertebral subluxation) and lack coordination of activities due the unsoundness of the tissue cell. Regardless, it is the innate law that maintains the material of the body alive (Prin. 21) through adaptation of information/F and E/matter for use in the body, so that all parts of the body will have coordinated actions for mutual benefit, if it is possible according to universal laws (Prin. 23, 24).

It is important for the student to understand that according to the principles of chiropractic's basic science, there can be interference in transmission of innate impulses caused by a vertebral subluxation. A vertebral subluxation always causes a lack of ease of the conducting nerve, which then alters the momentum of the transmission of the innate impulses, thus violating the principle of coordination (Prin. 29, 30, 31, 32). Therefore, it becomes crystal clear why the chiropractic objective is: The location, analysis, and facilitation of the correction of vertebral subluxations for a normal transmission of innate impulses.

ART. 88.   THE THIRD AFFERENT STEP OF THE NORMAL COMPLETE CYCLE FOR COORDINATION OF ACTIVITIES: IMPRESSION/RECODING

The impression of vibrations is the computed and coded effect of the receptor cells output motion from the instruction of the innate impulse within the cell's limitations (Prin. 24). It is the actual coded feedback within the innate field of the body part regarding its coordinated activities. It emanates from the tissue cell of the part's soundness and function. It is a salient feature of all the tissues of the body under the governance of the innate control. In the normal complete cycle for coordination of activities, this refers to the afferent transmission from any and every tissue cell of body part but does not refer to sense impressions (This will be expanded in further volumes). This salient feedback is an impression of the body part's output motion within its limitations. It is coded into through 100%/perfect integral adaptation from the innate law within the innate field and is transmitted through the afferent nerves. The innate field is literally a field. When a field is tickled or excited anywhere, it is experienced everywhere in that field. It is whole, complete, and non-discrete. Whatever activity goes on in the innate field fluctuates and sweeps across the whole field. The motion causing the vibration of the tissue cell is then impressed into a special impulse that will convey the impression of vibrations, which is coded by the innate law and is dependent on the limitations of the body part's receptor cell. It is also dependent on having received (or not having received) the correct instruction of the innate impulse. The receptor cell of the body part must also be sound metabolically to carry on its function coordinately.

ART. 89.   THE FOURTH AFFERENT STEP OF THE NORMAL COMPLETE CYCLE FOR COORDINATION OF ACTIVITIES: TROPHIC IMPULSE

A trophic impulse is a special impulse feedback coded by the innate law. It demonstrates the cell's metabolic soundness as well as its coordinative abilities. This feedback impulse is called a trophic impulse as opposed to an innate impulse which is information/F that has been characterized by the innate law with specific modal impression of vibrations of the metabolic and coordinative state of a body part's tissue cells as to whether it functions coordinately or not. A trophic impulse is transmitted through afferent nerves (See lexicon).

A trophic impulse is an impression of vibration. An analogy may help to make this clear. When you take a seat anywhere in a stadium to attend a rock concert, you position yourself within a complete unvariable and smooth sound circuit. It is the sound field of the stadium and is different from what you hear when the music begins. It makes no sound yet… Its cybernetic wave range is unvariable and does not change the microphone transmitter designed to produce sound frequencies through the vibration of its diaphragm or the loudspeaker driver designed to reproduce the sound frequencies through vibration of its own cone diaphragm. Both diaphragms do not vibrate and there is no sound. Then the leader of the band holds the microphone and begins to sing. The sound of his voice vibrates the diaphragm in the microphone transmitter changing (tickling or exciting) the electromagnetic field that forms fluctuating waves to be transmitted through the sound system of the stadium's cybernetic field. These fluctuating waves change the motion of the diaphragm and it vibrates within the loudspeaker device reproducing the microphone diaphragm vibration sounds from the voice of the lead singer. At no time do the vibrations of the singer's voice leave the microphone, or travel in cyberspace, as is popularly supposed by many persons who do not have much knowledge of electromagnetic field transmission. The voice that the listener hears is reproduced by "impression of vibrations," from the microphone diaphragm to the loudspeaker diaphragm, close to the listener in his seat, perhaps in the upper seats of the stadium hundreds of feet away from the singer.

ART. 90. THE FIFTH AFFERENT STEP OF THE NORMAL COMPLETE CYCLE FOR COORDINATION OF ACTIVITIES: AFFERENT NERVE

An afferent nerve is the conductor of trophic impulse from a body part (receptor) to brain (CPU) for feedback. It is a structural component of the bio-cybernetic feedback loop system used for coordination of activities. A trophic impulse is a coded impulse carrying specific modal impression of vibrations of the metabolic state of a tissue cell and its function that is either coordinated or not coordinated. The nerve-tissue cell consists of neurons that have many long cellular dendrites and axons that extend from their central bodies (Fig. 10). Afferent neurons transmit signals called trophic impulses from tissue cells to brain cells. Afferent neurons are neuron-transmitters of trophic impulses that conduct the output of the tissue cells of the body parts (including the brain cells) as feedback to the brain for central processing. This computation is ultimately for the continual coordination of actions of all the body parts for mutual benefit (Prin. 23).

Afferent nerves are comprised of tissue cells called neurons with a body, dendrites, and axons that act as feedback information highways to conduct trophic impulses between all the parts of the body, the spinal cord, and the brain. Afferent nerves are one-way neurons-transmitters as they only transmit trophic impulses, which are impressions of vibrations output, of the body part-receptor to the brain-CPU. In the normal complete cycle for coordination of activities, this does not refer to the special sense nerves. It refers to the communication that each individual body part (receptor) has with the brain (CPU) for the central processing of computation for coordination of activities. It is the feedback necessary for central processing to coordinate the activities of all the body parts for mutual benefit (Prin. 23).

Every tissue cell of the body of a living thing has an inborn organizing principle, called the innate law of living things (Prin. 20), which is an essential continuation of the universal principle of organization (Prin. 1). Afferent nerves are used to transmit trophic impulses communicating output feedback regarding the coordinative activities of the function of every body part and their metabolic condition (soundness). Philosophically, feedback must always be true to be a valid feedback, whether normal functions or abnormal functions. Therefore it is not possible for vertebral subluxations to interfere with transmission of feedback. Chiropractic is always about what is possible according to universal laws (Prin. 24). This is corroborated and verified anatomically as vertebral subluxations cannot impinge upon afferent nerve cell bodies since they run outside the spinal cord. Only efferent nerves can be impinged by vertebral subluxations (See Fig. 1). By infinitely gradual differences, some of these body parts are able to have better coordination of their actions than others due to their state of organization including their soundness, and the quality of the momentum of the innate impulses they received. The limitation of E/matter of those body parts is different. Because of this, any classification must be more or less arbitrary. For further study of efferent and afferent nerves, the student is directed to a 2021 presentation by Jaimar Tuarez.[24] The fact remains that the afferent nerves of bio-cybernetic output feedback are a vital aspect of the normal complete cycle for coordination of activities under innate control according to universal laws (Prin. 6, 24) to continually loop the input of innate impulses, through an interface processing to the output of body functions (Prin. 1, 10, 13, 20). Even if a sensory organ does not use trophic impulses we can use it as an analogy to help us better understand. For example, an odor sensed by the olfactory nerve, as a smell, will need to reach the olfactory interpretation center in the brain to be determined as sweet or pungent or sickening under the innate control. The same is true for the feedback of functional output of the body part. It must be transmitted to the brain-CPU for computation that will decode the trophic impulse for continual coordination of activities.

24. Tuarez, Jaimar. "The Difference between efferent and afferent nerves."
    https://neurotray.com/differencebetweenefferentandafferentnerves. Feb 2021

REVIEW QUESTIONS FOR ARTICLES 81 - 90

1. What is expression?

2. What is function as it pertains to the normal complete cycle?

3. What is primary function?

4. Name the nine primary functions.

5. What is coordination?

6. What is vibration as it pertains to the normal complete cycle?

7. What are impressions of vibrations?

8. Which is transmitted to the brain, vibrations or the impression of them?

9. What is the afferent nerve?

10. Can we anatomically point out the afferent nerves of the normal complete cycle for coordination of activities?

11. What is the name of the coded impulse conducted through afferent nerves and what is its function?

ART. 91. THE SIXTH AFFERENT STEP OF THE NORMAL CYCLE FOR COORDINATION OF ACTIVITIES: TRANSMISSION

Transmission is the carrying of impressions of vibrations to the brain as functional output feedback for central processing for coordination of activities. It is the afferent feedback of functional motion being conveyed to the brain to be computed by the innate law for coordination of activities. It is not a mechanical quivering of the nerve.

Transmission is just the same in afferent nerves as in efferent nerves. Impressions of vibrations are innate information/F recoded by the innate law. They are called trophic impulses because they carry not only functional output feedback but also metabolic output feedback from the body-part-receptor to the brain. Both the innate impulse and the soundness of the body part are necessary to carry normal functional motions. The metabolic state of the body part is intrinsic to the trophic impulse according to its limitations (Prin. 6, 24). Trophic impulses are coded by the innate law according to the level of organization of the body part, as manifested output, without breaking a universal law (Prin. 23, 24). The transmission of innate impulses (input-instructions) and trophic impulses (output-feedback) is accomplished in the same way. An impression is the computed and coded output feedback as the organized representation of the adaptability of the body part (Prin. 7, 18). This organized information/F, from the functional motion of the body part, is not transmitted as vibrations per se, but as a representation of the organization of the body part intrinsic to the vibrations, the trophic impulse.

ART. 92. THE SEVENTH AFFERENT STEP OF THE NORMAL COMPLETE CYCLE FOR COORDINATION OF ACTIVITIES: BRAIN CELL

The cells of the brain are neurons forming the central processing unit of the body under innate control for computing information/F into coded instructions for continual coordination of activities, if it is possible according to universal laws. The innate law is intrinsic to all tissue cells of the body of a living thing (Prin. 20) including the brain cells. The innate law adapts every single tissue cell of the body (Prin. 23). In this cycle for coordination of activities, the brain is the organ of innate control, operating as the central processing unit, where adapted and computed information/F (innate impulses) are processed into instruction input that will be conducted through efferent nerve transmitters to body parts receptors for functional output. The functional output is then computed within the body part and processed by the innate control as feedback output of its adaptability (trophic impulse). The feedback output then will be conducted through afferent nerve transmitters to the brain to be processed for coordination of activities. Note that the innate law always adapts, computes, codes and assembles information/F within the innate field, which is wherever the innate law acts, which is everywhere in each tissue cell in the body. It's analogous to the universal law of gravitation of planet earth, which is manifested in every particle of E/matter of planet earth.

ART. 93. THE EIGHTH AFFERENT STEP OF THE NORMAL COMPLETE CYCLE FOR COORDINATION OF ACTIVITIES: RECEPTION

Reception is impression (trophic impulses) that are manifested within the innate field of the central processing unit (brain) for coordination of activities. It is the arrival or receiving trophic impulses manifesting the functional motion output feedback. A brain cell is a tissue cell and as such is also a receptor cell in the same way as any tissue cell. The receiving process is then centralized within the innate field of the brain for continual coordination of activities.

ART. 94. THE NINTH AFFERENT STEP OF THE NORMAL COMPLETE CYCLE FOR COORDINATION OF ACTIVITIES: 100%/PERFECT INNATE REALM

It is the same plane of activity of the innate law, the 100%/perfect innate realm, as studied in the efferent half of the cycle (Art. 52).

ART. 95. THE TENTH AFFERENT STEP OF THE NORMAL COMPLETE CYCLE FOR COORDINATION OF ACTIVITIES: INTERPRETATION/ DECODING

Interpretation is the decoding of the impression (trophic impulse), the working out of the functional output feedback by the innate law. It is an innate process of conversion of the receiving content data from the feedback of the body part, which is communicated by the innate control to a processing device within the brain, capable of verifying the character of the trophic impulse and of assessing the coordinative ability of the body part, based on its functional motion. It is the decoding and adapting of the impression into computability, by the innate law, for coordination of activities. It changes from the material/immaterial output realm of motion of the body part to the only immaterial 100%/perfect innate processing realm.

When the unit of information/F from the impression reaches the brain it is decoded, processed, verified, and assessed according to the perfect processing of instructions contained within the 100%/perfect program of the innate law for the moment. This verification and assessment is a 100%/perfect innate processing and therefore it is in the innate realm. The process is just the reverse to that of transformation/ coding in the efferent half of the cycle. Here is one of many program flow charts at the receptor cell, under the innate control, demonstrating some of the computation steps of the innate process for coordination of activities:

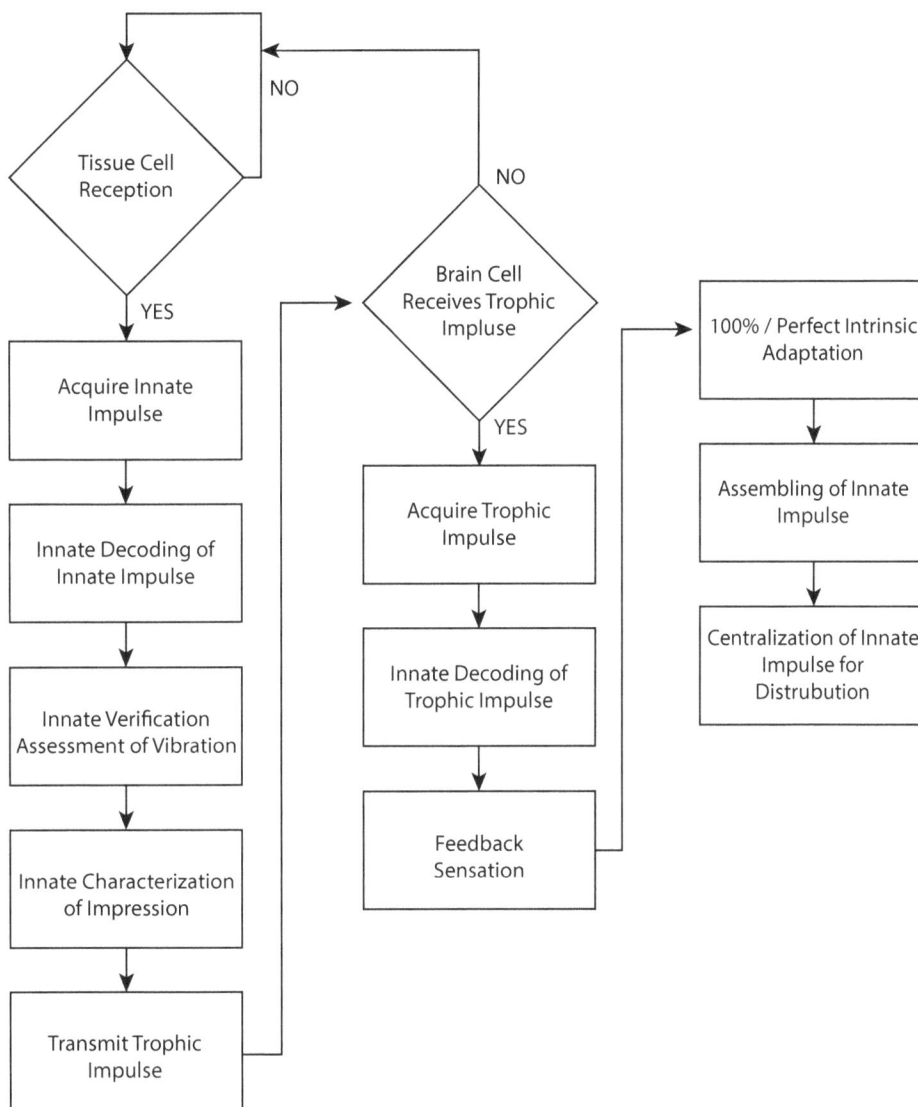

Fig. 12. Flow chart example of one tissue cell as receptor of innate impulses under the innate control, demonstrating some of the computation steps of the innate process for coordination of activities. This is true for every tissue cell of the body.

ART. 96. THE ELEVENTH AFFERENT STEP OF THE NORMAL COMPLETE CYCLE FOR COORDINATION OF ACTIVITIES: SENSATION

Sensation is a sense datum. It is the decoded feedback output of information/F from the functional motion of the body part that is leading to the construction of innate impulses for coordination of activities through 100%/perfect integral adaptation. It is a feedback output of converted instructive innate information/F, concerning the functional motion of a bit E/matter, impelled as trophic impulses, in time, for coordination of activities. It is a computation of the input of the decoded trophic impulses to be processed and prepared for 100%/perfect integral adaptation for coordination of activities.

Sensation is strictly an innate process or the output of an innate process. Since the innate law is 100%/perfect, the innate process of sensation is always normal (Prin. 22, 27). The feedback output of the functional motion may reveal lack of coordination of the part (due to a vertebral subluxation or for its not being sound), however the innate process of sensation is always normal (Prin. 27). As was mentioned in Art. 90, special sense organs transmit information/F to specific centers in the brain for processing of the sensation received for interpretation. It is the same process involved with the feedback output of the functional motion of a body part.

ART. 97. THE TWELFTH AFFERENT STEP OF THE NORMAL COMPLETE CYCLE FOR COORDINATION OF ACTIVITIES: INTEGRAL INNATE PROCESSING

Integral innate processing is the construction of innate impulse that is the sum total of the decoded feedbacks. It is the 100%/perfect innate control of all the computations of all the parts of the body for coordination of activities according to universal laws (Prin. 6, 24). Sensation is merely one bit (inforun); all the bits are necessary for complete and integral processing. Let us use an analogy. We read headlines on one news channel from the Internet stating that there has been a train derailment in New Jersey. The information conveys little at first and it is not until we read further particulars that we are able to begin to get the big picture. When we have read subsequent news broadcasts we are able to comprehend the situation adequately and understand the complete accident. Integral innate processing is entirely within the innate realm and involves all the decoded feedbacks moment by moment.

ART. 98. THE THIRTEENTH AFFERENT STEP OF THE NORMAL COMPLETE CYCLE FOR COORDINATION OF ACTIVITIES: INNATE LAW OF LIVING THINGS

It is the intrinsic organizing principle that computes and controls all living activities. It is the 100%/perfect normal software program governing every tissue cell of the body through its innate control. It is the same innate law studied in the efferent half of the cycle (Art. 50).

ART. 99. THE FOURTEENTH AFFERENT STEP OF THE NORMAL COMPLETE CYCLE FOR COORDINATION OF ACTIVITIES: 100%/PERFECT INSTANTANEOUS INTEGRAL ADAPTATION

It is the actual 100%/perfect program of innate computation functioning perfectly for every moment and circumstance to adapt information/F and E/matter for use in the body so that all parts of the body will have coordinated actions for mutual benefit (Prin. 23). It is the complete innate control maintaining the body alive within its limitations. It is the only function of the innate law.

It differs from adaptation in that 100%/perfect instantaneous integral adaptation is purely a non-material perfect organizing program designed by a universal intelligence capable of processing facts and counterfactuals (Art. 19, 21). It is the infinite organizing potential of unlimited potentialities and possibilities of the innate law. It is controlled through the innate field, which is a perfect operating system of unlimited possibilities and potentialities in order to compute non-material and material entities. It keeps living E/matter alive, if it is possible, according to universal laws (Prin. 22, 23, 24). On the other hand, adaptation is the physical representation of the 100%/perfect instantaneous integral adaptation and it is purely material. It differs from adaptability in that 100%/perfect instantaneous integral adaptation is the action of the program of instructive information/F of the innate law, while adaptability indicates the compliance of those instructive information/F by E/matter. It is the contrast between the ability of the organized activities and the action of the organizing principle. It is the function of information/F to unite the non-physical organizing principle with physical E/matter (Prin. 10). This instantaneous integral adaptation of information/F from the innate law generates instructions, which are the interface that unites the non-material to the material.

When the impression of the functional motion of the tissue cell is decoded in the innate field and manifests in the brain cell, the functional condition of the cells of the body part and the information/F exist there through the computation of innate processing based on their quantity, quality, and intensity. They are unified into a cooperative act to maintain coherence through the instantaneous integral adaptation under the innate control. They are coded for coordination of activities of that moment. These codes are instructions that are in the form of innate impulses to meet the challenges of the internal and external environment of all the parts of the body for that moment. 100%/perfect instantaneous integral adaptation is purely non-material, non-discrete. It is intrinsic to the 100%/perfect program capable of unlimited computation of infinite possibilities and potentialities designed by a universal intelligence. Therefore, all internal and external environmental challenges of any moment are engaged perfectly within the limitations of E/matter. This instructive computation under innate control takes place in the innate realm which in non-material. Any computer software program is instructive data meant to process input and to transform it into output. Chiropractic concerns itself with the link that interface with the non-material input and the material output.

For example, a person eats a garden salad. The body must adapt to the sudden intake of nutrients that was not there a moment ago. This experience is unique and has never existed before, in so far as the food is different, the person's metabolism of this particular moment is different, their body weight is different, their age is different, their body temperature is different, their blood pressure different, it's a different day, etc… They may have had many garden salads before, but it was not this one at this moment. Every time the person eats is a unique experience at that moment. Every situation must be dealt with according to every manifestation of motion of everything going on internally and externally at this particular moment. The next moment will bring a new set of challenges. Thus, we see that there is a continual change in the construction of innate information/F.

There is a unique process of innate computation of construction that is dependent upon these environmental challenges. Immediately, the innate law will adapt all the information/F and all the parts of the body, in that particular moment, through instantaneous cooperative interoperability of infinite functioning motions, for coordination of activities, according to the environmental circumstances of that particular moment. This instantaneous cooperative interoperability process of computation occurs within all the cells of the body simultaneously (Fig. 12). It is a very fine working of the law of systematic change. Unlike a laptop computer, every part of the body of a living thing is vital for every single moment for coordination of actions for mutual benefit. There is a great variation and interoperability of instructive information/F for the coordination all the activities of all the parts of the body. That is why it is called: 100%/perfect instantaneous integral adaptation.

The students are advised to get this principle well in mind, for thereupon depends their understanding of many subjects based upon it. Remember that the flow of innate instructive information/F to a body part is never constant but always changing according to each moment. The expression 100%/perfect connotes perfection of change.

The normal complete cycle for coordination of activities is an organized flowchart of some of the steps leading to the transmission of the conducted information/E. Should any of the body part receptors fail in their functioning, some other parts, somewhere, will lack. Imperfection of the flow of innate impulses of the working of the law of continuous supply and computation, due to limitations of E/matter anywhere in the body, will cause a lack in the experience of the moment at all levels. Vertebral subluxations interfere with the working of that law.

A
Start

Enzymes: special proteins that control each of the interrelated reactions of metabolism, as well as the steps of DNA replication and protein synthesis

Peptide bond: Dipedptide (2 bound ammino acids) Polypeptide (many linked) Protein (hundreds of amino acids linked)

Dehydration Synthesis: the removal of a water molecule in order to join two smaller molecules into one larger one

Anabolism: the buildup of larger molecules from smaller ones

B
Metabolic Reactions

Catabolism: the breakdown of larger molecules into smaller ones.

Hydrolysis: decomposition of carbohydrates, lipids and proteins and the splitting of a water molecule

Breakdown of fat, protein and nucleic acid molecules

C
Control of Metabolic Reactions

Activation Energy: the amount of energy required to start reactions that enzymes lower

Substrate: the only chemical a specific enzyme can act on

Active Site: the part of the enzyme molecule that binds to a substrate

Catalysis: the acceleration of metabolic reactions

Some enzymes are active until they combine with a Coractor: a non-protien component

May combine with organic molecule called a Coenzyme

D
Energy for Metabolic Reactions

Energy: the capacity to change or move matter

Oxidation: process where cells "bum" glucose molecules

Cellular Respiration

Gylcosis: The 6 carbon sugar is broke down in the cytosol into two 3 carbon pyruvic acid molecules with a net gain of 2 ATP and the release of high-engery electrons

Citric Acid Cycle

Electron Transport Chain

E
Metabolic Pathways

Metabolic pathway: a sequence of enzyme-controlled reactions

Rate-limiting enzyme: as it's name implies, it is an enzyme that regulates metabolic rates within a pathway

Aerobic Respiration

Although most energy is lost as heat, almost half is captured in the form of high energy electrons so that the cell can store it through synthesis of ATP

Anaerobic Respiration

F
DNA (Deoxyribonucle Acid):

DNA: molecules that hold information in the form of genetic code

Adenine, Tymine, Cytosine and Guanine make up the genetic code (more accurate to state that by "information" we mean the effects of these chemicals reacting)

Genes: the portions of DNA molecules that contain the genetic infromation, hence the adjective "genetic"

Genome: all of the DNA in a cell

DNA replication goes on during the interphase of a cell

Gene that is transcribed and translated into a protein is expressed

G
Protein Synthesis

Genetic Code: the correspondence of gene and protein building block sequence

Transcription: the copying of DNA information into RNA which can exit the nucleus

Codons: three base synthesis in mRNA that represent amino acids

Translation: the process of protein synthesis

Transfer RNA (tRNA): RNA that correctly aligns amino acids

Anticodon: the three nucleotides in tRNA

RNA uses Uracil instead of Thymine

mRNA (aka messenger RNA) is the type of RNA capable of carrying infromation out of the cells nucleus

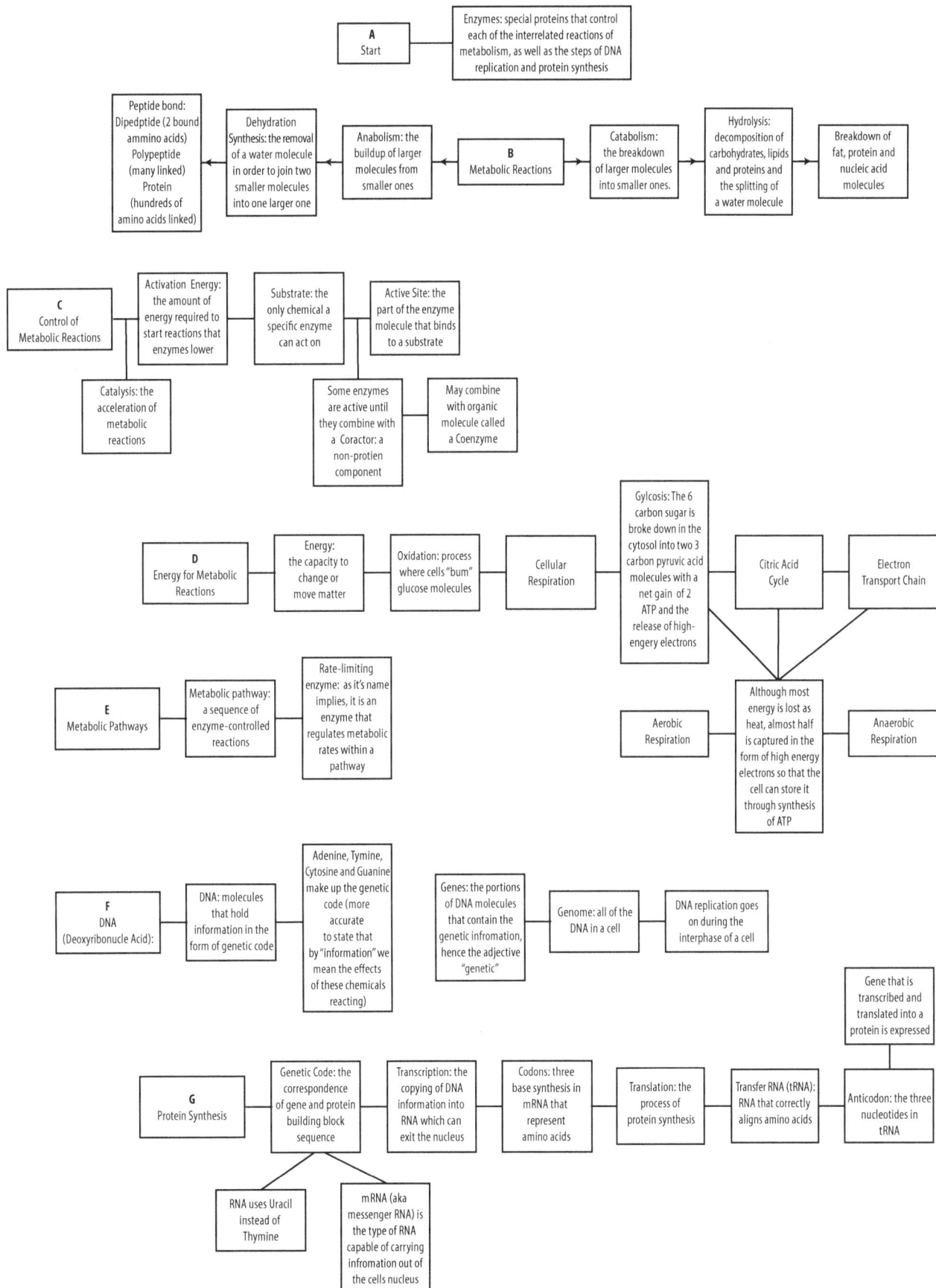

Fig. 13. One of many flow charts of continual, simultaneous, systematic change of multiple cellular functions simultaneously processed by the innate law.

ART. 100. THE FIFTEENTH AFFERENT STEP OF THE NORMAL COMPLETE CYCLE FOR COORDINATION OF ACTIVITIES: UNIVERSAL PRINCIPLE OF ORGANIZATION

It is the 100%/perfect infinite organizing principle of the universe, designed by a universal intelligence, maintaining everything in existence. The universal principle of organization is the beginning and the ending of the normal complete cycle for coordination of activities. The normal complete cycle for coordination of activities is a description of some arbitrary steps involved in the coordination of activities of the parts of the living vertebrate body and as such, it has no beginning and no end. It is a continual cycle.

As chiropractic moves forward through its second century, all chiropractors, together and without condemnation, will acquire new information and construct new knowledge. They will harness a greater understanding of chiropractic and they will continue to develop its philosophy, science and art for future generations to come.

ART. 101. CONTINUATION OF THE NORMAL COMPLETE CYCLE FOR COORDINATION OF ACTIVITIES

The normal complete cycle for coordination of activities is a narrative summary of what happens between cause and effect and effect and cause. The list of the 31 steps is the conventional outline of the narrative. It is imperative to remember that the normal compete cycle for coordination of activities has no beginning and no end except that which we ascribe to it. It continually runs and is infinitely congruent with the initial principle of chiropractic's basic science (Prin. 1).

Having arrived at this point, we can now present the chiropractic narrative.

The Merriam-Webster Dictionary defines *narrative* as:

> Something that is <u>narrated</u>: STORY, ACCOUNT

The Chiropractic Narrative

The universal principle of organization, designed and programmed by a universal intelligence, is intrinsic to all E/matter and is continually organizing information/F through an unlimited program of infinite computations that supplies all the properties and actions of E/matter, through the configuration and velocity of electrons, protons and neutrons to maintain it in existence. The expression of this organizing principle, through E/matter is the chiropractic meaning of existence. Therefore maintaining the existence of E/matter is necessarily the interface of the organizing principle and E/matter; it is the link between the two. It is the organized information/F (instructive information) that unite the organizing principle and E/matter. The information/F of this universal organizing principle instructs the structure of organic E/matter toward a higher level of complexity of its manifested existence; it is called, the innate law of living things. The innate law is the essential continuation of the organizing principle for living things.

The purpose of the innate law of living things is to maintain the material of the body of the living unit alive. The innate law does this by adapting universal information/F and E/matter, organized by the universal principle, (which are manifested by physical laws that are unswerving and un-adapted, and have no solicitude for structural E/matter), so they can be used in the body for coordinated action and mutual benefit of all body parts. This work of adaptation of the innate law is 100%perfect, non-discrete and is entirely in an innate realm. For this reason, the instructive information/F of the innate law never injures or deconstructs the tissues. The 100%/perfect computing program of instructive information/F of the innate law is distinct from the programming of information/F of the universal principle because it adapts them and assembles them for use in the body of a living thing to maintain it alive. This innate adaptation of information/F takes place within the innate field. Regarding coordination of activities, information/F emanates from the brain cell as conducted information/F that is then centralized for transmission.

This assembling of universal information/F to be adapted by the innate law is called characterization. It is the coding of innate information/F, which is the interface between the organizing principle and E/matter, occurring within the innate field, intrinsic to every cell of the body, for they eventually have definite form and purpose. The operating system is the innate field (which is non-discrete) controlled by innate law, which uses a definite unit, the brain cell (which is discrete) for coordination of activities. From the brain cell as a unit, the innate law controls a unit of E/matter for coordination of activities of body parts (including the brain cell). This is how the non-material is united to the material. The non-physical information/F interfaces with physical E/matter when the innate law characterizes and transforms this information/F into a definite unit, for a given tissue cell of a body part, for a given moment. For coordination of activities, this non-material information/F when it is characterized and transformed under innate control becomes an instructive information/F that is both non-material and material emanating from the material brain cell. It is specifically coded instructions, providing input/output operations under innate control, which is setting E/matter into action for coordination of activities. It is called innate impulse. This specialized neurological brain system is necessary to first, centralize the already assembled innate impulses, and then to conduct their instructive information to the different parts of the body. The departure of the innate impulse from the brain cell is called propulsion/conductivity.

For the innate impulse to be conducted, from brain cell to tissue cell, requires action. The conducted information/F of the innate law operates through or over the nerve system. That which has efferent direction (CPU to receptor) and which conducts the innate impulse is called the efferent nerve. Since physical conductors can suffer interruption in their conductivity, the conducted innate information/F can suffer interference with its conduction: and that is the justification for the existence of chiropractic. This comparison is the basis of our theory that the innate impulse is half material and half non-material, and therefore, the conductivity momentum of the material nerve is subject to the same laws as any other material conductor. The conveyance of the innate impulse over the efferent nerve is transmission. This specialized neuronal circuitry with specialized atomic elements with particular configuration and velocities is the route the innate impulse travels to the tissue cell where it is received. Subsequently, the 100% integral notion of computed and decoded instructive information/F of the innate law as to what the cells of the body part should be or how it should act in the moment comes to pass. That which was only non-physical innate information/F now becomes a physical fact. It shows by its very character that a 100%/perfect program computed the form or the action and this evidence of the perfect programming is called expression. Expression is the coming forth through E/matter, the showing of the intelligent programming of infinite computations, moment to moment. Things which show this are said to be alive and such expression is called life. The character of this action is determined by the character of the system adapted by the innate law to express its instructive information/F for coordination of activities. Therefore the purpose or the action of this system, which is the tissue cell of the body part, is function.

The function of E/matter is to express instructive information/F. In the tissue cell, which is a specific kind of E/matter, the specific instructive information/F of the innate law are expressed in a specific manner by a genetic device driver which is a specific material constructed for the particular kind of expression (perhaps the mitochondria). The prompt and correct action of all the tissue cells of the body part being actuated by the specific instructive information/F of the innate law, in coherence with all the other parts of the body, is called coordination. In this we see the working of the law of cause and effect, and that every process requires time. To perform its function, the tissue cell has motion, both molecular and as a whole cell. This movement is called vibration, which is a specific configuration and velocity of the subatomic particles of the cell under innate control. These vibrations give off signals, which are impressed upon specialized nerves as a form of physical impulse called impression. These impressions are coded in the form of trophic impulses and are transmitted over the afferent nerve. This transmission is similar to transmission in the efferent half of the cycle, for the information/F are similar with the exception that, philosophically, feedback must always be true to be a valid feedback, whether normal functions or abnormal functions.

When the feedback reaches the afferent brain cell, it is received much in the same manner as the tissue cell receives, for the brain cell is also a tissue cell. When this innate information/F, in the form of trophic impulse, has reached the brain cell, it is immediately within the innate realm being decoded and interpreted in the innate field by the innate law. The outcome of this act of decoding and interpretation under the innate control is a feedback sensation, which is a computation of the trophic impulses. When this feedback has a sum of computations, the resulting data is processed and the functional condition of the cell is determined under innate control and this is named integral innate processing, which is a clear representation of the state of the tissue cell. This integral innate processing can be nothing but 100%/perfect organization. Perfection in the body, of course, is the innate law of living things, which bespeaks intelligence. When the innate law processes the state of the tissue cells of the body part in the innate field, information/F are coded and assembled by the innate law to coordinate its actions controlling its adaptability to its environmental conditions within its limitations. The innate process of doing this is called instantaneous integral adaptation, which is the 100%/perfect continual assembling and construction of information/F by the innate law to instruct the tissue cells of the body part for a specific moment. The origin of this continuous supply and computation from which the innate law carries its instructive information/F is the universal principle of organization designed and programmed by a universal intelligence.

REVIEW QUESTIONS FOR ARTICLES 91 - 101

1. What is afferent transmission?

2. What is an afferent brain cell?

3. What is afferent reception?

4. What is interpretation?

5. What is trophic impulse?

6. What is sensation?

7. Where is sensation as considered in the normal complete cycle for coordination of activities?

8. What is integral innate processing?

9. What is instantaneous integral adaptation and where does it take place?

10. Is the flow of innate impulses constant or changing?

11. What expression means the same as the law of systematic change?

12. Be able to give a complete summary of the normal complete cycle for coordination of activities.

ART. 102. REVIEW OF PRINCIPLES

As a conclusion of Volume One, the student should return to the introduction and study carefully the principles of chiropractic's basic science. Learn to give, verbatim, the 33 principles. Review Article 22, 23, and 24 and be able to answer the review questions of those three articles.

Proceed to Volume Two.

BIBILOGRAPHY VOL 1:

1. Strauss, Joseph. "The Green Book Commentaries, Vol. XIV (1927) Chiropractic Text Book" Levittown, PA: Foundation for Advancement of Chiropractic Education. (2002) p. 17

2. Palmer, B.J., "The Science of Chiropractic, Its Principles and Philosophies." 4th Ed., Davenport, IA: The Palmer School of Chiropractic - Chiropractic Fountain Head. (1920) p. 12

3. Stephenson, R.W. "Chiropratic Text Book" (Vol. XIV) Davenport, IA: The Palmer School of Chiropractic (1948) p. xiii

4. Gold, Reginald. Sherman College Course Philosophy 801 Notes, Spartanburg, SC (1976) p. 5

5. Gelardi, Thom. "Sherman College of Chiropractic 76-78 Catalog" Spartanburg, SC: Sherman College of Chiropractic (1976) p.12

6. Lessard, Claude. "Timed Out: Chiropractic." Self-published, Claude Lessard D.C. (2022)

7. Stephenson, R.W. "Chiropratic Text Book" (Vol. XIV) Davenport, IA: The Palmer School of Chiropractic (1948) p. xviii

8. D.D. Palmer, editor Palmer, B.J. "The Chiropractic Adjuster." Davenport,IA: The Palmer School of Chiropractic (1921) p. 316

9. Stephenson, R.W. "Chiropratic Text Book" (Vol. XIV) Davenport, IA: The Palmer School of Chiropractic (1948) p. xxi

10. Kuhn, Thomas S. "The Structure of Scientific Revolution." Chicago, IL: The University of Chicago Press. (1962)

11. Kuhn, Thomas S. "The Structure of Scientific Revolution." Chicago, IL: The University of Chicago Press. (1962) p.12

12. Lessard, Claude. "Timed Out: Chiropractic." Self-published, Claude Lessard D.C. (2022) p. 144-148

13. Wilson, A.D., Golonka S. "Embodied cognition is not what you Think it is." Front Psychol. 2013; 4:58 Published 2013 Feb 12.

14. "Brain Basics: The Life and Death of a Neuron." https://www.ninds.nih.gov/health-information/public-education/brain-basics/brain-basics-life-and-death-neuron#:~:text=A%20neuron%20has%20three%20basic,sends%20messages%20from%20the%20cell June 2023

15. "The Cellphones of the 1980s." techcentral.co.za/the-cellphones-of-the-1980s/191544 Jan 2015.

16. "Steve Jobs debuts the iPhone." history.com/this-day-in-history/steve-jobs-debuts-the-iphone. Published Aug 2012.

17. Bellis, Mary. "What is Electricity?" thoughtco.com/what-is-electricity-4019643 Sept 2018.

18. MillerKeane Encyclopedia and Dictionary of Medicine, Nursing, and Allied Health. Seventh Edition. Saunder, and imprint of Elsiver, Inc. 2003 p.1652

19. MillerKeane Encyclopedia and Dictionary of Medicine, Nursing, and Allied Health. Seventh Edition. Saunder, and imprint of Elsiver, Inc. 2003 p. 1277

20. MillerKeane Encyclopedia and Dictionary of Medicine, Nursing, and Allied Health. Seventh Edition. Saunder, and imprint of Elsiver, Inc. 2003 p. 1451

21. MillerKeane Encyclopedia and Dictionary of Medicine, Nursing, and Allied Health. Seventh Edition. Saunder, and imprint of Elsiver, Inc. 2003 p. 1145

22. MillerKeane Encyclopedia and Dictionary of Medicine, Nursing, and Allied Health. Seventh Edition. Saunder, and imprint of Elsiver, Inc. 2003 p. 1684

23. MillerKeane Encyclopedia and Dictionary of Medicine, Nursing, and Allied Health. Seventh Edition. Saunder, and imprint of Elsiver, Inc. 2003 p. 220

24. Tuarez, Jaimar. "The Difference between efferent and afferent nerves." https://neurotray.com/differencebetweenefferentandafferentnerves. Feb 2021

CURRICULUM VITAE
DR. CLAUDE LESSARD

- B.S. Limestone College, Gaffney, S.C. 1977

- Doctor Of Chiropractic Degree, Sherman College Of Straight Chiropractic (S.C.S.C), Spartanburg, S.C. 1977

- Internship, S.C.S.C. 1977

- Recipient Of The B.J. Palmer Chiropractic Philosophy Distinction Award, S.C.S.C. 1977

- Diplomate Of The National Board Of Chiropractic Examiners

- Certified For Preliminary Professional Education #C35301, Commonwealth Of Pennsylvania

- Commonwealth Of Pennsylvania License #DC-1702-L

- Co-Founder And Charter Member Of ADIO Institute Of Straight Chiropractic 1978

- Student Referral Counselor, ADIO I.S.C. 1978-1981

- Assistant Professor Of Chiropractic Philosophy, ADIO I.S.C. 1978-1980

- Co-Developer of The ADIO Analysis 1978

- Administrative Dean Of ADIO I.S.C. 1979-1980

- Associate Professor Of Chiropractic Technique, ADIO I.S.C. 1980-1981

- Director Community Health Center, ADIO I.S.C. 1980-1981

- Member Chiropractic Life Fellowship Of Pennsylvania

- Member Of The Federation Of Straight Chiropractors Organization (F.S.C.O.)

- Graduate Of Church Ministry Program, St. Charles Borromeo Seminary 1983-1987

- Certified Myotech Examiner

- Chiropractor Of The Month Award, Markson Management Services, 1988

- Chiropractor Of The Year Award, Markson Management Services, 1992

- Post Graduate Course Of Study In Applied Spinal Biomechanics From The Aragona Spinal Biomechanic Engineering Laboratory, Inc. 1992

- Chiropractor Of The Year Award, Quest Management Systems, 1993

- Member Of The Distinguished Board Of Regents, S.C.S.C. Since 1993

- Member Of Parker Chiropractic Resources Foundation

- Chair And Co-Author Of "Spirit Of '76", S.C.S.C. 1996

- Founder Of Clients Association For Chiropractic Education (C.A.C.E.), 1997

- Licensed Private Pilot, Single Engine Airplanes Land, 1998

- Founder Of Lessard Institute For Chiropractic Clients, 1998

- Recipient Of The Spirit Of Sherman College Of Straight Chiropractic Award, 1999

- Licensed Pilot, Instrument Airplanes, 2000

- Author Of "Chiropractic.... Amazing Isn't It?" 2003

- Chiropractor Of The Year, S.C.S.C., 2006

- Motion De Felicitations, Ville De Ste. Anne De Beaupre, Resolutions 5553-09-06., 2006

- Pulstar Examiner, 2008

- Translation Of "Chiropractic…Amazing Isn't It?" In French, 2008
- Translation Of "Chiropractic…Amazing Isn't It?" In Spanish, 2009
- Autor Del Libro "Quiropraxia No Es Asombrosa?" 2010
- Auteur Du Livre "La Chiropratique, Incroyable N'est-Ce Pas?" 2012
- Author Of Blue Book "A New Look At Chiropractic Basic Science" 2017
- Autor Del Libro Azul "Una Mirada A La Scienca Basica Quiropractica" 2019
- Keynote Speaker At Sherman College Of Chiropractic International Research And Philosophy Symposium, 2019
- Author Of "Chiropractic, Amazing Isn't It- Workbook" 2020
- Author of Blue Book "Timed Out: Chiropractic" 2022
- Autor Del Libro Azul "Quiropractica Reseteada" 2023

www.ingramcontent.com/pod-product-compliance
Lightning Source LLC
Chambersburg PA
CBHW040140200326
41458CB00025B/6331